It Takes a Village

The Role of the Greater Community in Inspiring and Empowering Women to Breastfeed

Edited by
Paige Hall Smith, MSPH, PhD
and
Miriam Labbok, MD, MPH, IBCLC

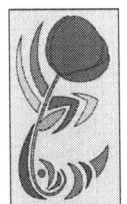

Praeclarus Press, LLC
©2015 Paige Hall Smith & Miriam Labbok. All rights reserved.
www.PraeclarusPress.com

Praeclarus Press, LLC
2504 Sweetgum Lane
Amarillo, Texas 79124 USA
806-367-9950
www.PraeclarusPress.com

All rights reserved. No part of this publication may be reproduced or transmitted in any form, or by any means, electronic or mechanical, including photocopy, recording, stored in a database, or any information storage, or put into a computer, without the prior written permission from the publisher.

DISCLAIMER

The information contained in this publication is advisory only and is not intended to replace sound clinical judgment or individualized patient care. The author disclaims all warranties, whether expressed or implied, including any warranty as to the quality, accuracy, safety, or suitability of this information for any particular purpose.

ISBN: 978-1-939807-24-3

©2015 Miriam Labbok & Paige Hall Smith. All rights reserved.

Cover Design: Ken Tackett
Acquisition & Development: Kathleen Kendall-Tackett
Copy Editing: Chris Tackett
Layout & Design: Todd Rollison
Operations: Scott Sherwood

It Takes a Village is based on the presentations at the 8th Breastfeeding and Feminism International Conference, March 21-22, 2013, Sheraton Chapel Hill, Chapel Hill, NC

Editors

Paige Hall Smith, MSPH, PhD

School of Health and Human Sciences

University of North Carolina at Greensboro

- Associate Professor, Public Health Education
- Director, Center for Women's Health and Wellness

Miriam Labbok, MD, MPH, IBCLC

Department of Maternal and Child Health, Gillings Global School of Public Health

University of North Carolina at Chapel Hill

- Founding Professor and Director, Carolina Global Breastfeeding Institute

Introduction

This volume results from the 8th Breastfeeding and Feminism International Conference (BFIC) held March 20-21 at the Sheraton Hotel in Chapel Hill, North Carolina. The conference was jointly sponsored by the Center for Women's Health and Wellness at the University of North Carolina at Greensboro and the Carolina Global Breastfeeding Institute at the University of North Carolina at Chapel Hill. This conference has brought together academic scholars with policy makers, health care professionals, activists, communications specialists, students, and others who are interested in the sociocultural, economic, health, and political impacts on, and of, women's infant feeding decisions since 2004. Since its inception, the BFIC has focused attention on the need for public health and medical approaches to breastfeeding to go beyond promoting health to include serious consideration of the realities of women's lives, which are complicated by economic, political, and social inequities in gender, race, and sexuality. We are publishing this volume

It Takes a Village

in order to make the information and ideas presented at the BFIC more widely available.

Our theme for the 2013 conference was *It Takes a Village: The Role of the Greater Community in Inspiring and Empowering Women to Breastfeed*. This theme reflects the ancient idea that a healthy and wise next generation is a social good. The caring and rearing of children is best recognized as a responsibility—and a joy—to be shared by all of us, not to be apportioned only to mothers. It is critical that our social structures, our social norms, and our laws and policies reflect the worth and dignity of all of us regardless of our age, race, sex, gender, sexuality, religion, or abilities.

Lactation, as a gendered biological trait, and breastfeeding, a gendered form of caregiving, presents unique challenges to the village construct, however. As a gendered biological process, breastfeeding is something mothers, not villages, do. Breastfeeding requires mothers and babies to be together, a biological necessity that is difficult for most, and impossible for many mothers, given the structures and policies affecting how we work, caregive, and live today. We are constantly challenged to make it possible for all women to both breastfeed and achieve full economic, social, and political equality of opportunity, treatment, and status. This is why it actually does "take a village" to feed a baby: women who breastfeed need the active support of families, communities, institutions, and governments.

Introduction

Our collective work at the Breastfeeding and Feminism International Conference, by highlighting the importance of women's equality and rights at home, at work, and in the community, is designed to be a valuable contribution to the global public-health breastfeeding promotion, protection, and support efforts. The chapters in this volume are organized to summarize the different ways that our villages can support and empower women as they seek to breastfeed. As these chapters discuss, we need to consider the parameters of our villages across the social ecology; reduce inequalities in gender, race, and ethnicity; listen to and build upon women's experiences; help women integrate mothering and breastfeeding with employment; engage whole communities; improve birth facility and professional support; increase access to human milk; and expand and improve media support for breastfeeding.

We believe that a published volume of conference papers should reflect the presentations at the conference, hence the papers here have not been substantially edited; however, the authors were limited in terms of length and figures. Although, some conference papers are missing from these proceedings by the author's choice, a total of 40 papers are presented here.

Rutgers University Press published an edited book based on presentations at the 2010 conference (Smith, Hausman, & Labbok, 2012), and we partnered with the *International Breastfeeding Journal* to publish a thematic series of nine articles based on the 2007 conference (Published August 4, 2008). Our goal is to publish a volume reflecting the themes of all subsequent BFICs to share the rich presentations with a broader audience.

More information about the conference can be found at www.breastfeedingandfeminism.org, or on Facebook at "Breastfeeding and Feminism International Conference."

We would like to thank the staff and students affiliated with both the Center for Women's Health and Wellness, and the Carolina Global Breastfeeding Institute, for their support and hard work over the years. In particular, we would like to acknowledge the following for their support in producing this volume: Melanie Pringle, 2014 Graduate Research Assistant, Center for Women's Health and Wellness; Thea Calhoun-Smith, Business Services Coordinator; Carolina Global Breastfeeding Institute; and Quirina Vallejos, 2013 Graduate Research Assistant, Center for Women's Health and Wellness, School of Health and Human Sciences, University of North Carolina at Greensboro.

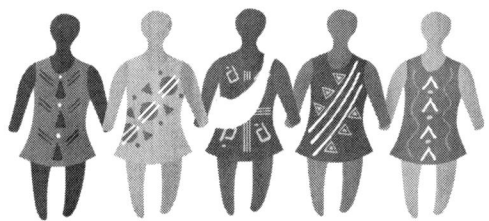

Table of Contents

Introduction   5

Chapter 1
Considering the Village   17

It Takes a Village: Latest Thinking on Community-Based Participatory Approaches to Behavior Change   17

The Global Village: Do Women Live There? A Critical Look at Global Approaches to Breastfeeding Promotion, Protection, and Support   23

Does it Really Take a Village? Self-efficacy and Social Support Theory and Research   32

> Breastfeeding and the Status of Women   36
>
> The Inadequate Breast: Medical and Social Origins of Breastfeeding Myths   44

Chapter 2
Eliminating Inequalities in Gender, Race, and Ethnicity   53

> The Welfare State and the Breastfeeding Worker   53
>
> Breastfeeding Equity: Summary of a Concept Analysis   59
>
> Milk and Motherhood: Breastfeeding and "Good Motherhood" Among African American Women in the South   65
>
> Undoing Institutional Racism in Perinatal Support Organizations: First Steps for Eliminating Racial Inequity in Breastfeeding Support   72
>
> Mothers and Others: An Intervention with Promise for Improving Breastfeeding Outcomes among African American Women   79

Differences in Early Breastfeeding Experiences and Outcomes in Spanish versus English-Speaking Latinas from the Early Lactation Success Study Cohort of First-Time Mothers   85

Chapter 3
Building on Women's Experiences   97

Brown Mamas Breastfeed—An Analysis of African American Women's Breastfeeding Experiences Shared through an Online Blog Project   97

Early Infant Feeding Practices among Mothers with High Body Mass Index   103

Breastfeeding Narratives among WIC Participants in Alamance County, North Carolina   110

The Challenges of Nighttime Breastfeeding in the U.S.   117

The Challenge of Late Preterm Birth on Realizing Breastfeeding Intentions   123

*Expectant Moms Respond to "Risk" and
"Benefit" Language in Breastfeeding
Promotion: Evaluating the Impact of
Language on Efficacy*   136

Chapter 4
Helping Women Integrate Breastfeeding And Employment   143

*Advancing the Breastfeeding-Friendly
Campus: Cultivating University Climates can
Inspire Change in the Community*   143

*Development of Indicators to Evaluate the
Presence of Worksite Breastfeeding Supportive
Policies, Benefits, and Environments*   150

*Establishing an Employee Lactation Program
in a Large Municipal Health Agency.*   156

Chapter 5
Engaging Communities in Support of Breastfeeding Women   165

*Empowered Communities Ensure
Breastfeeding and Good Nutrition of Mothers
and Infants*   165

*Evaluation of Breastfeeding Peer Support
in a Rural Area: What Works for Young,
Disadvantaged Women and Their Babies?*   172

From Bottles to Breasts in Rural Haiti   180

*Associations between Frequency of
Interpersonal Contact Opportunities and
Exclusive Breastfeeding Coverage in USAID's
Child Survival and Health Grants Program*   185

Chapter 6
Improving Birth Facility and Professional Health Care Support   195

Lactation Consulting and the Role of Family-Centered Care in Professional Breastfeeding Support   195

Application of the Relational Theory to an Academic Program in Maternal Child Health Lactation Consulting: The Transformative Power of Learning   204

Low-Income Women's Experiences with Breastfeeding and Lactation Support: A

> Program Evaluation of a Community Home
> Visitation Service   221
>
> "We Just Have This One Breastfeeding
> Brochure" (Sponsored by Enfamil): Exploring
> Breastfeeding Resources and Agenda-Setting
> in Pediatrics' Offices, WIC, LLL, and the
> Community Hospital   225
>
> Growing Breastfeeding Advocates among the
> Next Generation of Nurses   229
>
> The Role of Growth Pattern Interpretations on
> U.S. Women's Breastfeeding Decisions   234
>
> The Role of Postnatal Unit Bassinet Types on
> Enabling Early Breastfeeding   239

Chapter 7
Increasing Access to Human Milk   249

> Increasing the Use of Donor Human Milk:
> An Assessment of Knowledge, Beliefs, and
> Practices Among Key Stakeholders in North
> Carolina   249

*The Gift of Milk: How Altruistic Milk Sharing
Practices Empower Women* 256

Donor Human Milk: Past, Present and Future 263

Chapter 8
Expanding and Improving Media Support for Breastfeeding 273

*Chasing the Numbers: Measuring Social
Influences on Breastfeeding* 273

*Mediating Mother Support: Social Networks,
Online Discussion, and Breastfeeding Support* 280

*A Look at the World Breastfeeding Week
Public Announcement Videos in Quebec, "Je
l'ai fait ... / I did it ..." and "Allaitement c'est
glamour /Breastfeeding is Glamour"* 286

*Portrayals and Representations of Infant
Feeding Practices in Primetime U.S. Television
Media: A Discourse Analysis* 291

*Media Reactions to Breastfeeding: Reactions to
Recent Headlines* 296

It Takes a Village

    Defeating the Formula Death Star, One Tweet at a Time: Using Social Media to Advocate for the WHO Code   299

Contributors   309

References   323

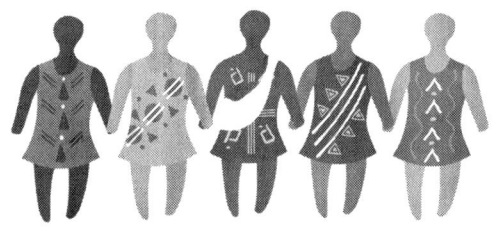

1

Considering the Village

It Takes a Village: Latest Thinking on Community-Based Participatory Approaches to Behavior Change

Geni Eng and Miriam Labbok

In sharing "latest thinking" on community-based participatory approaches to behavior change in the field of public health, it might be useful to start with the genesis of such thinking, and how it has influenced the trajectory of my own work and thinking. Today, I will share with you why it takes a village to be an equal partner with researchers and practitioners in order to ensure the conditions for people to be in good health, and also discuss why this is so relevant in the South and for UNC, Chapel Hill. For ex-

It Takes a Village

ample, the first Department of Public Health Education in a School of Public Health was chaired by Dr. Lucy Morgan at UNC, Chapel Hill from 1942 to 1966. Having conducted assessments of health issues and concerns of communities across the State, she recognized the need for public health professionals who are African American. Faced with a university that would admit only White students, Dr. Morgan had her faculty drive to North Carolina College for Negroes in Durham (later North Carolina Central University) to train the State's first African American health educators. Moreover, she required students from both institutions to conduct field training together in both Black and White communities.

In the early 1960s, Greensboro, North Carolina entered headlines, and Civil Rights history in the U.S., with the 1960 lunch-counter sit-in efforts by A&T University students to advocate for the rights of African Americans to be served by eating establishments. In 1963, hospital desegregation was at the center of the case of Simpkins versus Moses Cone Memorial Hospitals. The history and success of this case was documented in an article published in the *Annals of Internal Medicine* in 1997. This case was recognized as the landmark case that led to the elimination of segregated hospitals nationwide. The spirit and passion of these historic civil rights movements in Greensboro motivated subsequent residents to continue the struggle for equality–especially in health care.

From 1968 to 1985, Dr. Guy Steuart chaired the Public Health Education Department and instituted, a 21-month field training in community assessment and community development, bringing together faculty trained in anthropology, psychology, and other social sciences. In 1964, Bill Darity earned a PhD in Health Education, becoming the first African American to receive a doctoral degree from the UNC Graduate School and SPH. Subsequently, the faculty, too, expanded to include well-known scholars, such as Godfrey Hochbaum, JoAnne Earp, Brenda DeVellis, Allan Steckler, Tony Whitehead (African American anthropologist), and eventually John Hatch (African American health educator), Ethel Jackson (African American health educator), and Joyce Kramer (American Indian sociologist).

Let's examine community-based participatory research approach using the metaphor of the bowl. I am Chinese American and in my culture, the bowl is seen as a duality. A bowl's dimensions and materials that form it represent boundary, border, control, and limitation. However, what makes the bowl useful is the empty space inside. If there were no empty space, it would not be a bowl. The bowl's empty space represents room, freedom, and opportunity. By joining these contradictions, something unexplainable or magical happens—the resulting whole is very different from the two original sources. There is a similar duality in the joining together of the field of public health and the CBPR approach, which strives to bring together health agencies, universities, and communities as insiders and outsiders to function and be productive as equal partners.

It Takes a Village

A community provides care through sociability, influence, Mutual Aid, an organizational Base, Reference Groups, Status Arena, and Referral. A community produces citizens. In contrast, the service delivery system seeks to solve problems, and acts by *providing* goods and services that are standardized and always the same—consistent quality we can count on. The service delivery system *produces* clients. By seeing these as a duality, rather than a dichotomy, we can more effectively form research partnerships to enhance health equity and community competence.

Although training in providing culturally competent care is intended to raise an individual service provider's awareness of racial/ethnic/tribal disparities, this approach does not move us toward assessing and addressing the less visible realities of implicit bias in our own system or gaining tools to modify or create structures at the system level to increase transparency of and accountability for equity in race-specific patient outcomes. We must learn from history about constructed racial oppression and granted White privilege, encourage culture sharing on internalized racial oppression and internalized White supremacy, distinguish prejudice, oppression, and racism, and analyze power dynamics within our society and gatekeeping.

The People's Institute for Survival and Beyond, a non-profit, anti-racism training organization out of New Orleans, developed a two-day Undoing Racism Training. It teaches concepts and strategies related to community organizing and systems change–while fostering relationship building through various activities. It has allowed our Greensboro Health Disparities Collaborative to be more OPEN with one another. We are not worried about being "politically correct," but CLEAR about any issue we discuss. This strengthens our understanding of one another, which makes it EASIER to talk about difficult issues of historic oppression, why my people are categorized as "mongoloid," for example.

Prejudice ... damaging because it denies a person his or her individuality

Oppression exists when:

1. The oppressor group has the power to define reality for themselves and others,

2. The target groups take in and internalize the negative messages about them, and

3. Members of both groups are socialized to play their roles as normal and correct.

Community participation in decision-making may be seen as a ladder of what might happen when the system's way and the community's way are brought together as a dichotomy, rather than as a duality. The results are Non-Participation and Tokenism at the most bottom rungs. To avoid these, all must have a voice and hold the power to insure that a community's views will not be eclipsed, or made invisible, by well-known hierarchical structures and patterns

It Takes a Village

of how decisions are made. At the higher rungs of the ladder is Partnership, at which decision-making power is delegated and made transparent to the citizens of the community, along with ensured accountability through citizen veto power and citizen control.

Today, our Greensboro Health Disparities Collaborative is working on five-year, community-based participatory research (CBPR) project, funded by the National Cancer Institute, called Accountability for Cancer Care through Undoing Racism and Equity (ACCURE). Our goal is to test a system's change intervention at two cancer centers on improving quality and completion of care for early stage breast and lung cancer, narrowing the racial gap between Black and White patients, and enhancing patient self-reported health status, health care utilization while reducing medical mistrust and perceived racism. We are applying the People's Institute Undoing Racism language, set of concepts, and assumptions to inform the intervention that provides transparency and increases accountability for racial equity in cancer care. We sincerely hope that the ACCURE Partners will clearly demonstrate the strengths of the duality, and hence, the power of the Bowl.

The Global Village: Do Women Live There? A Critical Look at Global Approaches to Breastfeeding Promotion, Protection, and Support

Miriam Labbok

Global policies and international conventions tend to view breastfeeding through the framework of Human Rights. According to the Convention on the Rights of the Child, affirmed by nearly every country worldwide—except the United States—all parents should be informed of the importance of breastfeeding to their children's health, and every baby has the right to the best start on life. Therefore, if breastfeeding is important for health, and every baby has this right, then every baby has the right to be breastfed.

In this construct, for every right, there is a duty-bearer, responsible for supporting that right; clearly, mothers are the primary duty-bearers for breastfeeding. However, it is vital to note that the rights construct does not stop there. For every primary duty-bearer, in this case, the mother, who is responsible for the rights of another, that duty-bearer has the right to the support of secondary and tertiary duty-bearers, in fact, her entire society, to enable her to fulfil her responsibility. In other words, no mother has the responsibility to breastfeed a child unless she is completely—in every possible way–supported to make the decision and to succeed with her intentions to breastfeed. Hence, no woman can be "expected" to breastfeed unless she is "enabled"— by culturally sensitive, unbiased information and complete social, economic, and clinical support—to decide to breastfeed, and is then given every and all the social, clinical, political, and economic support she may need to achieve her breastfeeding goals.

Where do men fit into this construct? In the rights construct, it is their duty to fully and actively support optimal feeding in their families and workplaces, and in *all* the acts they do in relationship to women and children, and other current and future fathers. However, to fulfil this duty, they must ensure that women are enabled to express all of their own needs related to breastfeeding success, and that all those needs are met.

Expressing This in Action

How is this expressed in action? In many different ways. Let's consider one example of an effort to support breastfeeding. At a recent World Breastfeeding Conference held in New Delhi, the slogans were, "Babies need Mom-made, not man-made! Come join the fight. Let's protect every feeding mother," with a picture of a fist, a broken feeding bottle, and a well-dressed mother smiling down on her sleeping baby in her arms. In a short play, the formula company representative was indicated by a large U.S. dollar sign.

I invite you to consider each of the three slogans and the use of the U.S. dollar sign from the perspective of a feminist, a woman, a breastfeeding mother, or whatever perspective drew you to this discussion. Please observe your emotional and intellectual reactions to the slogans and images.

- Come join the fight! (illustrated with a fist)

- Babies need Mom-made, not man-made! (illustrated with a broken feeding bottle)

- Let's protect every feeding mother! (illustrated with a photograph of a lovely mother and sleeping child)

- (A photo of skit that "villainized" Nestlé by having the representative wearing a U.S. dollar sign.)

The comments during the conference included concern with the use of fighting words with a picture of a passive woman, use of a fist, as this could be associated with abuse, combative rather than supportive of women, and one comment that breaking a bottle is not supportive of breastfeeding, as many women must express milk to be fed by other means. There was also considerable concern that the photograph evoked the "Good Mother" discourse, in which the good is externally defined. Finally, there was concern expressed that Nestlé is a Swiss company but that, globally, the U.S. is often targeted for its perceived commercialism.

Given the venue and the slogans of the World Breastfeeding Conference, it may not be a surprise that the panels and speakers were predominantly men. There was only one woman speaker in the opening session and only one in the closing session. Is it men's roles to define women's needs, or is it men's role, among others, to invite women to express their needs and then to support them?

It Takes a Village

To help us understand why this has occurred in the global breastfeeding arena, it may be helpful to look at the major global policies related to breastfeeding and also examine their origins. First, it may be important to understand whether any policy or convention supports positive or negative rights. Positive rights are those that guarantee a right for a specific population, while negative rights are those that prevent someone from denying another's right. For example, *positive rights* are enumerated in the UN Convention on the Rights of the Child, ratified by the United Nations in 1989, which calls for the "highest attainable standard." This is the construct used in most nations around the world: You must ensure access to health for all. *Negative rights* appeared in the U.S. Constitution: The Bill of Rights articulates negative rights in that Congress is prohibited from passing laws that restrict freedoms. In the U.S., we have predominantly negative rights: You cannot deny another the right to health. One could argue that the Code of Marketing and the CEDAW also guarantee negative rights.

Do you view the slogans in yet another light when considering them from the viewpoint of positive and negative rights? Comments included that the reaction was informed by this construct, but that the initial reactions were not dependent on this intellectual construct.

Most global agreements or policies are presented in either the positive or the negative, in part due to the motivation behind them and the purpose brought to the fore by their supporters. After the International Labor Organization called upon countries to legislate a minimum number of weeks guaranteed paid maternity leave in the early part of the 20th century (a positive right), perhaps the first major policy related to breastfeeding that followed was the International Code of Marketing of Breast-milk Substitutes. An organization called the International Baby Food Action Network (IBFAN) was formed by consumer protection groups in 1979 in support of the development of a Code of Marketing to reduce false and misleading marketing of human milk substitutes. This was to protect women against false and misleading advertising, but initially did not include specific support or promotion for breastfeeding. Over the years, the scope of IBFAN has been expanded to include manufactured children's foods, reaching beyond the scope of the Code, continuing the support as a negative right.

The World Health Organization's Code was ratified in 1981, the same year that the Convention on the Elimination of All Forms of Discrimination Against Women (CEDAW) was ratified. It may be important to note that this convention condemns discrimination and calls for equality, but does not address creation of equity. It also is stated in the negative: women cannot be discriminated against in seeking equal opportunities, information, and choices, including in formal and non-formal sectors. Similarly, the Code also condemns a negative: false and misleading advertising to the public by formula manufacturers. Neither of these calls for women in leadership nor offers support for women themselves to achieve equity nor calls for women's voices.

Instead, they both are designed to fight the social and commercial powers that might misuse or abuse women.

These efforts to fight misuse and abuse of women are most welcome, of course. While these movements were sparked by women, their leadership, which included rights activists, consumer's union and researchers, were occasionally male-dominated arenas. IBFAN, for example, is a network of 273 member groups in 168 countries, including consumer organizations, health workers associations, parents' groups, and diversity of organizations in the social justice movement. Groups, such as women's groups, mother-to-mother groups, and feminist groups do not come to the fore.

Consider whether "Consumer Protection" serves as a useful framework for breastfeeding support?

The discussion that followed included positives and negatives of basing our discourse and actions on this framework and positives and negatives of having male leadership for breastfeeding action.

However, when it was time to consider children, in the late 1980s, the Convention on the Rights of the Child supports positive rights for children, rather than highlighting what should not be done to them. Just for a moment, let us consider the practical effect of subordinating women's rights to children's rights. This may be seen to reinforce women's disempowerment, i.e., "the best interests of the child," could conflict with women's right to full equality.

However, as stated above, the woman is not subordinate, but rather a duty bearer with rights that must be respected if she is to be asked to breastfeed.

The difference between positive and negative rights as discussed above may seem subtle, but there is definitely a difference in message and required action. Perhaps it is most obvious in that whenever there is a meeting on the rights of the child, youth are particularly invited to have a voice. It is not as clear that meetings on the Code of Marketing invite the voice of women or women's groups, per se, even these are the individuals protected by this Code. Rather, as noted, the call is to fight for babies: "Babies need Mom-made, not man-made! Come join the fight." And we outsiders are called upon to protect only those mothers who are doing what we are calling upon them to do: "Let's protect every feeding mother." But what is it that women NEED in order to decide to breastfeed and to succeed with breastfeeding?

In 1990, both the CRC and the Innocenti Declaration, which followed in the same year, are stated in terms of positive rights. CRC states that the child has the right to the healthiest start on life. This offers that the parents' decision-making should be governed by the best interests of the child. The Innocenti Declaration calls upon countries to ensure that every woman lives in a country in which the Code is legislated and the government has oversight of two women's rights: the right to breastfeeding-supportive maternity care and guaranteed paid maternity leave, as well as paid workplace accommodation. Clearly, in this case, the promotion of women's rights and promotion of children's rights are complementary goals. There is always the potential for tension between women's and children's rights, but if we consider again that no woman is required to act upon such children's rights unless the rest of her society is fully responsive to her rights as related to this duty, there is complementarity, rather than tension.

Worldwide gender inequality and inequity remain despite all of these efforts, whether you consider the lower income of women compared to men in the U.S., or the percent of parliamentarians in all countries, or the low female literacy rates in South Asia, Africa, and elsewhere, and so on. Women's decision making power impacts on her ability to fulfill parental duties. There is less low weight among children when women's decisions are empowered; this relationship holds even after controlling for education, income, sanitary conditions, etc. One study concludes that in South Asia, making women's status equal to men's would reduce rates of malnutrition from 49 to 37%—a 24% reduction!

It is of interest that all of these policies and conventions place substantial obligations on the "state," or country. CEDAW defines maternity as a societal function. The CRC's requires states to "render appropriate assistance to parents … in the performance of their childrearing responsibilities." Clearly, these conventions may serve as grounds to require state support maternity and childcare.

Considering the Village

So let us return to the question of men's roles in these constructs. The *obligations placed on both parents* by the CRC, and CEDAW can be entry points for promoting discussion about the roles of fathers in childrearing in a manner that challenges traditional gender norms. Ensuring that women's and children's rights are mutually reinforcing requires *confronting social assumptions* about the appropriate roles of both women and men, and emphasizing community and state responsibilities for care of children.

Near the end of the session, the audience was informed of the outcome of the World Breastfeeding Conference (http://info.babymilkaction.org/update/update45page4) and encouraged to chat amongst themselves to consider these issues from the perspective of the global community: 1) Which approach do you feel will have more impact in the long run in enabling women to succeed in optimal feeding: evidence-based advocacy, women's rights, children's rights, or consumer's rights? And, 2) How do you think various audiences in North America and beyond would react to these slogans?

All are invited to continue to consider these issues and to continually seek to increase women's profile in decisions concerning her own body and roles, and her empowerment within the global village.

Thank you for all you do every day to support women and their decisions to breastfeed.

Does it Really Take a Village? Self-efficacy and Social Support Theory and Research

Deborah McCarter-Spaulding

Ask a new mom her plans for infant feeding, and you may get the answer "I'll breastfeed if I am able." As a nurse and IBCLC, "if I am able" is puzzling and disturbing. Why would a woman anticipate that she would not be able to do what her body is uniquely designed to do? I believe the answer lies in the concept of self-efficacy.

Self-efficacy is part of Bandura's Social Cognitive Theory, and is defined as a belief in one's capabilities to organize and carry out a course of action required to produce a particular (specific) result (Bandura, 1997). How a person perceives their ability to be successful will influence what they choose, how much effort they will expend, how long they will persevere in the face of challenges or problems, as well as how they feel about what they are doing.

Four sources inform efficacy beliefs. The first is **enactive mastery**, a.k.a., personal experience. The second is **vicarious experience**, such as observing role models who are attempting or accomplishing the task/goal at hand. The third is **verbal persuasion**, or what one is told about their ability to succeed (e.g., with feedback and encouragement). The fourth source of efficacy information is **physiological and affective states**, which include emotional and physical feelings and sensations. Much of this efficacy information comes from a person's social environment; for example, having someone to help facilitate a positive experience in attempting a behavior or task. The social environment (the village) also may provide role models as well as education, coaching, and emotional support–or it can work against a positive perception of self-efficacy if the information received from the social network is negative and disaffirming.

Health Efficacy and Health Behaviors

Self-efficacy theory provides insight into how people make changes in health behaviors. Self-efficacy perceptions influence whether a person chooses to adopt a behavior, how much they will persevere in the face of challenges, and ultimately how well they will maintain the change or health behavior. The choice to breastfeed a baby can be understood as a health-promoting behavior, the success of which may be influenced by a mother's breastfeeding self-efficacy.

Breastfeeding self-efficacy can then be defined as a mother's belief that she will be able to organize and carry out the actions necessary to breastfeed her baby. Such actions may include getting the infant to latch comfortably, establishing a sufficient milk supply, managing the psychological and social aspects of incorporating breastfeeding into one's lifestyle, as well as coping with various challenges, and establishing a support network, to name just a few.

Research studies have demonstrated that higher levels of breastfeeding self-efficacy predict both a longer duration and a more exclusive pattern of breastfeeding, and these results are consistent in diverse groups of women (Creedy et al., 2003; Dennis, 2003; Gregory, Penrose, Morrison, Dennis, & MacArthur, 2008; McCarter-Spaulding & Gore, 2009; Mossman, Heaman, Dennis, & Morris, 2008; Torres, Torres, Rodriguez, & Dennis, 2003; Wutke & Dennis, 2007). Research has also demonstrated that positive social support can contribute to breastfeeding success, particularly when provided by the father (Wolfberg et al., 2004) and/or the grandmother of the infant (Grassley & Eschiti, 2008), but also when provided by peers (Kaunonen, Hannula, & Tarkka, 2012) and professionals (Hannula, Kaunonen, & Tarkka, 2008).

Breastfeeding Self-Efficacy and Social Support

In research study conducted in a sample of Black women (McCarter-Spaulding & Gore, 2012), both breastfeeding self-efficacy and social support were analyzed as potential influences on breastfeeding outcomes. Consistent with previous research, higher levels of breastfeeding self-efficacy predicted a longer duration and more exclusive pattern of breastfeeding. In contrast, social support did not predict either the duration or the pattern of breastfeeding, as might have been anticipated. However, higher levels of social support predicted higher levels of breastfeeding self-efficacy. This suggests that social support could be understood as a source of efficacy information.

These results support both self-efficacy and social support theory. Both variables are modifiable, which provides

Considering the Village

a theoretical foundation for planning evidence-based interventions designed improve breastfeeding outcomes, such as initiation, duration, and exclusivity. The "village" can be an influence on each of the four sources of efficacy information.

For example, as personal experience is the most potent source of efficacy information, any intervention that supports a positive and affirming first experience of breastfeeding will enhance a new mother's self-efficacy. This could include interventions, such as facilitating skin-to-skin contact immediately after birth (Bramson et al., 2010), or nurses providing practical advice in a caring and supportive manner (Phillips, 2011). In the framework of self-efficacy theory, this support enhances success in first experiences of breastfeeding, providing enactive mastery. But it also decreases anxiety, which modifies the affective state, another source of efficacy information. Mothers with previous successful experiences with breastfeeding have higher levels of self-efficacy, making this first experience a critical source of information for subsequent experiences. In addition, experienced successful breastfeeding mothers make great role models!

Vicarious experience, or role modeling, informs a person's perception of self-efficacy, especially when there is little prior experience (e.g., first-time breastfeeding), and is most effective if the role model available is perceived as being similar (Bandura, 1997). Facilitating peer groups as well as professional support similar in socioeconomic or marital status, racial/ethnic identity, employment, or other demographic variables will allow the "village" to provide accessible vicarious experience and enhance self-efficacy.

Verbal persuasion is most effective if it is realistic and believable, and provided by someone whose judgment is valued. Such people in the village may be professionals, peers or family. Such encouragement and support works best in conjunction with other sources of efficacy information. As people also rely on the physiological and affective states for efficacy information, encouragement can help to decrease anxiety, which in turn will enhance breastfeeding self-efficacy. Managing physical discomfort (Strong, 2011), as well as addressing postpartum depression (Field, 2010), will also support higher levels of breastfeeding self-efficacy.

Having a theoretical basis for interventions promotes excellence in clinical practice as well as research. Such sound scholarship can provide a framework for policy changes, research funding, and practice improvement. It supports what the village of breastfeeding advocates has understood intuitively, and anecdotally, and has the potential to improve the breastfeeding experience and outcomes for all women.

Breastfeeding and the Status of Women

Paige Hall Smith and Quirina Vallejos

Social changes over the past decades have led to dramatic changes in women's roles. Particularly impressive are the increases in women's participation in the paid labor market. Since 1975, there has been a 78% increase in the mothers of young children who are employed and, although women still are not paid as well as men, there has been an increase in women's income absolutely and relative to men. Women's increasing participation in the paid labor market has increased women's economic, political, and social status. Women now have more income and economic and economic authority, more women hold political office and there is a persistent gender gap in how women and men vote. Additionally, although in recent years there have been renewed assaults on women's reproductive freedoms, women still have more control over their reproductive lives than they did in the 1970s.

As women gain more wealth, autonomy, power, and control from their occupational role, and less from their maternal role, it is hypothesized that many maternal-related caregiving activities, such as breastfeeding, might decline. However, recent theoretical and empirical research suggests higher status of women may be associated with higher rates of breastfeeding initiation, exclusivity, and duration. Indeed, epidemiological research at the individual level consistently finds a strong relationship between breastfeeding and status in that breastfeeding is positively associated with education and income. Smith (2012) presented a theoretical argument that articulates how continued gender inequities in labor, power, and social relationships undermine women's abilities to breastfeed by: limiting women's access to resources and opportunities; reducing their power over these resources, as well as over their own bodies; sexualizing women's bodies and breasts as objects of male desire; and by increasing the stress women face when seeking to navigate multiple roles that cross-gendered norms and spaces.

No research has been conducted that looks at the effects of macro-level indicators of the status of women on rates of breastfeeding initiation, exclusivity, and duration. The purpose of our study was to examine the impact that the status of women at the state level has on five breastfeeding outcomes using state-level data from the 50 states plus the District of Columbia.

Methodology

Data Collection

We created an SPSS data set based on publicaly available data. Data on five breastfeeding outcomes (ever breastfed, exclusive breastfeeding at 3 months, exclusive breastfeeding at 6 months, breastfeeding at 6 months, and breastfeeding at 12 months) were taken from the 2012 CDC Breastfeeding Report Card. Data for the 2012 report card were derived from the 2010-2011 National Immunization Survey, which utilized data on births in 2009 (*http://www.cdc.gov/breastfeeding/data/reportcard.htm#Outcome, accessed January 29, 2013*). Hence, 2009 became our target year. Because it is important that our indicators of the status of women precede or reside

Economic Security	Economic and Social Autonomy	Reproductive Rights	Political Participation
• More women employed • Low gender gap in income • Higher income • More women in professional and managerial positions	• Access to health insurance • More women with a college education • More women living above poverty • More women business owners	• Prochoice legislation • Less restrictive reproductive choice legislation • Access to abortion • Access to contraception	• More women voting • More women holding political positions

Table 1 - Conceptualizing the Status of Women

concurrent with breastfeeding outcomes, all our indicators for the status of women were for the year 2008 or 2009.

Our conceptualization of the status of women at the state level was taken from the categories and measures used by the Institute for Women's Policy Research (IWPR) in their Status of Women reports. These state-level indicators fall into four well-accepted categories: employment and earnings; social and economic autonomy; political participation; and reproductive rights (See Table 1). The IWPR publishes annual reports on some, but not all, of the indicators of status of women. When available we used IWPR reports on the status of women indicators for the year 2009. For those indicators that were not available for 2009 from IWPR, we identified comparable data from the same sources as those used by the IWPR for the year 2009. Assignment of states to one of four regions was based on census bureau designations for West, Midwest, South (west and east) and Northeast (U.S. Census Bureau).

Data Analysis

Bivariate analysis, using SPSS v. 21 (IBM, 2012), revealed that the various indicators of the status of women (SOW) were highly correlated with each other. For this reason, we combined them into global measure of SOW (GSOW) that was used for our analyses. In testing our main variables for linearity we found that, although in many cases, the relationships between the composite GSOW and breastfeeding outcomes were somewhat curvilinear, the relationships

Breastfeeding Outcomes

Spearman's Correlation

Predictors	Ever breastfed		BF at 6 mo.		BF at 12 mo.		Exclusive BF at 3 mo.		Exclusive BF at 6 mo.	
	Rho	Sign	Rho	Sign	Rho	Sign	Rho	Sign	Rho	Sign
SOW	.481	.000	.532	.000	.490	.000	.389	.004	.404	.003

Regression

	T	Sign	T	Sign	T	Sign	T	Sign	T	Sign
SOW	3.697	.001	4.029	.000	3.463	.001	2.316	.025	2.338	.024
Region										
NE	2.922	.005	2.878	.006	3.095	.004	2.746	.009	1.907	.063
MW	5.132	.000	4.516	.000	3.373	.001	3.808	.000	3.244	.002
W	6.368	.000	4.823	.000	5.046	.000	5.659	.000	5.043	.000

Table 2 - Associations between the Status of Women (SOW), Region and Breastfeeding (BF) Outcomes: Results from correlation and regression analyses (N=51)

were sufficiently linear for use in multiple regression analysis. We determined the association between the GSOW and breastfeeding outcomes using Spearman's Correlation, and between region of the country, GSOW, and breastfeeding outcomes using regression. For analysis purposes we created one variable for each of the four regions: Northeast (NE); Midwest (MW), West (W) and South (S). Each region variable is coded so that it is compared against the other three regions; in this analysis South is left out, and therefore acts as the standard against which the other regions are compared.

Results

In bivariate analysis, the SOW and region of the country were significantly associated with each other and with all breastfeeding outcomes. Analysis of the correlation coefficients indicated that the strength of the association between GSOW and the breastfeeding outcomes lessened as the duration and exclusivity lengthened (Table 2). After controlling for differences among regions of the country, GSOW remained significantly associated all breastfeeding outcomes.

Conclusion and Discussion

This is the first study to assess the impact that the status of women at the state level has on breastfeeding initiation, duration, and exclusivity. Our study indicated that state-level breastfeeding rates are higher in states where women, collectively, have more economic security, personal autonomy, control over their reproductive decisions, and more political power. This finding lends support to the argument that the empowerment of women is linked to their infant feeding decisions in ways that favor breastfeeding over infant formula. This connection is not given much attention in policies and programs designed to support women's empowerment or breastfeeding (Van Esterik, 1989).

On the positive side, this relationship suggests that many women are able to find ways of integrating their productive and reproductive lives, and that there are opportunities for the development of alliances between individuals and groups interested in women's empowerment and those interested in breastfeeding. On the flip side, it suggests that other groups of women, those with less economic, social, and political status, find it more difficult to reconcile the different roles and responsibilities in their lives. This suggests the need for breastfeeding advocates, practitioners, and researchers to seek common ground and alliances with those concerned with poverty, the wages and benefits for the working poor, health access, and child welfare. Policies and programs that seek to advance women's empowerment and breastfeeding-friendly environments are potentially synergistic and worthy of further attention from the research and practice communities.

It Takes a Village

The Inadequate Breast: Medical and Social Origins of Breastfeeding Myths

Jacqueline H. Wolf

While "it takes a village" to inspire and empower women to breastfeed, it also takes a village to discourage generations of women from breastfeeding. More than a century of medical advice and cultural change have colluded in the United States to convince generations of women that lactation is an unreliable body function.

One hundred and twenty years ago, when women did not breastfeed, their primary explanation was that they didn't have enough milk. Today, women who initiate breastfeeding, but quickly turn to formula, offer the identical explanation. For well over a century, mothers have doubted the ability of their bodies to produce satisfactory milk, and doctors and the community at large have reinforced that distrust (Wolf, 2000).

There are many contemporary examples of this phenomenon, both on the individual and public level. One week after a colleague of mine gave birth to her first baby, her pediatrician advised her to supplement with formula because her baby had insufficient weight gain. He also instructed her to pump a few ounces of her own milk and let it stand in a glass jar. He explained that if after two hours, her milk did not have a half-inch of fat on top, then her milk was not fatty enough to assure adequate weight gain. When women

Considering the Village

hear this kind of authoritative (but in reality, nonsensical) advice from their physicians, they share with friends and family how difficult breastfeeding can be.

There are also public examples of this collective doubt that breasts "work." The Federal Emergency Management Agency, the American Red Cross, and the U.S. Department of Agriculture, for example, have developed a brochure titled, *Food and Water in an Emergency*. This brochure mentions breastfeeding in the context of emergency. But this is its pronouncement on breastfeeding: "Nursing mothers may need liquid formula, in case they are unable to nurse" (FEMA brochure). The presumption, both medical and cultural, is not that a breastfeeding mother is able to provide food for her baby in an emergency without worry, as opposed to the formula-feeding mother who might not have anything to feed her baby in the face of a Katrina-like disaster. Rather, the assumption is the opposite—that the human breast is destined to founder, but formula can be counted on to save babies in emergencies.

Our tendency to think of lactation as an unreliable body function began in the last quarter of the 19th century when mothers began to complain of their milk's inadequacy. In 1886, one typical mother sent a letter to *Babyhood* magazine's "Mother's Parliament" column to explain why she had turned to bottle-feeding with each of her children. She wrote: "the bottle was like food from heaven to the poor, starved little beings, who were weary and well-nigh spent with the struggle to sustain life on the meager and innutri-

It Takes a Village

tious milk which nature had unkindly provided" (Mother's Parliament, 1886).

Physicians voiced similar worries, offering theories in newspapers and women's magazines to explain the phenomenon. Isaac Abt, a Chicago pediatrician, predicted in a 1904 *Chicago Tribune* column that because women inherit from their mothers the inability to lactate that "the nursing function" in humans would gradually disappear (Abt, 1904). This belief—that breastfeeding was a disappearing function in human evolution—was soon echoed nationwide at child welfare conferences (Levenstein, 1983).

Abt's explanation was one of many. One of Abt's contemporaries, Thomas Rotch, a Harvard pediatrician, theorized that the sedentary lifestyles of middle- and upper-class urban mothers decreased the water and increased the solids in their milk. He advised exercise, telling lactating women to walk one to two miles a day to "reduce the albuminoid percentage" in "very bad" or "very rich" milk (Rotch 1890, 1896). Theories espoused by other doctors included the "overcivilization" and "overeducation" of women. Physicians speculated that urbanization had created an artificial environment detrimental to women's reproductive functions. Those who offered "overeducation" as an explanation speculated that because girls were now in school during puberty, their maturing bodies were competing with their brains for energy and their brains were winning, dooming future procreative abilities (Clarke, 1873).

Normal Human Milk and Bad Human Milk Caused by Lack of Exercise

	Normal Mother's Milk	Mother's Milk Causing Infant to Vomit Mother not Exercising	Mother Walking 2 Miles Daily, But Has Blisters from Wearing French Shoes Infant Still Vomiting	Mother Walking 2 Miles Daily Wearing Good Shoes Infant Doing Well
Fat	4.00%	3.05%	0.65%	3.34%
Sugar	7.00%	6.10%	5.35%	6.30%
Proteids	1.50%	3.89%	3.82%	2.61%
Ash	0.15%	0.16%	0.18%	0.16%
Solids	12.65%	13.20%	9.90%	12.41%
Water	87.35%	86.80%	90.10%	87.59%
Total	100.00%	100.00%	100.00%	100.00%

Table 3 - Adapted from Rotch, Thomas Morgan. (1896). *Pediatrics the hygienic and medical treatment of children.* Philadelphia: J. B. Lippincott Company, p. 191.

Of all his contemporaries, Rotch spent the most time devising ways to remedy women's inadequate milk. In his text, *Pediatrics: The Hygienic and Medical Treatment of Children*, he claimed to demonstrate that the content of human milk varied according to women's proclivities. Failing to exercise, or wearing uncomfortable French shoes, according to Rotch, could cause a mother to produce milk that would make her baby sick (see Table 3).

Rotch's explanations for why individual mothers produced "bad" milk gave rise to the invention of formula. Given that the content of breast milk could theoretically change, depending on a host of influences, over which mothers had little control, he proposed "formulas" as a solution. In the 1890s, Rotch coined the word "formula" in relation to infant food referred to the use of complex mathematical formulas to dictate the percentages of fat, protein, and milk sugar in individual babies' artificial food.

Mothers took these "formulas," written by pediatricians like prescriptions, to urban milk laboratories, where chemists created the indicated mixture. Formulas called for changes in minute fractions of one percent of a particular ingredient in cows' milk. Rotch based each mathematical formula on a number of variables, including (but not limited to) an infant's age, weight, appearance, ability to digest (and there were dozens of these conditions, "protein digestion weak" is one example), energy output, and the texture, color, and odor of a baby's stools (Rotch, 1896, 1901, 1904). As one doctor commented at the time, pediatrics was becoming "terrifyingly like higher astronomy" (Brennemann, 1938).

Physicians' efforts to mitigate the effects of babies' consumption of cows' milk were understandable—mothers' changing infant feeding habits had prompted a public health disaster. If mothers did not breastfeed in that era, babies consumed raw cows' milk. And before pure food laws, pasteurization, and refrigeration, cows' milk was a deadly alternative to human milk (Wolf, 2001).

One public health poster headlined *Mother's Milk for Mother's Babe, Cow's Milk for Calves* illustrated the problem. The poster depicted a long tube placed at one end on a cow's udder, and on the other in a baby's mouth. Between the two, the tube snaked through a muddy barnyard, milk cans baking in the hot sun, an unrefrigerated railroad car, and, just before landing in the infant's mouth, a front stoop with flies buzzing around an uncapped bottle. The poster advised, "To lessen babies' deaths, let us have more mother-fed babies" (Bulletin, 1911). (See Figure 1.)

Why did mothers fail to breastfeed when the consequences were so dire? Mothers' complaints of inadequate milk were likely correct, although infant-feeding schedules were the probable cause, not physiological milk insufficiency as physicians suspected.

In the 17th century, infant feeding advice had been appropriately vague. As a typical 1672 childrearing guide recommended: "As to the time and hour, it needs no limits, for it may be at any time, night or day, when he hath a mind" (Salmon, 1994). By the late 19th century, however, mothers had learned to feed their babies according to the mechanical clock. Before industrialization, Americans lived by natural rhythms—the rising and setting of the sun and when the cows needed milking. Thus, Americans having to deliver grain barrels at a precise time in order to meet the incoming train represented enormous cultural change. In adopting infant-feeding schedules, mothers were preparing their babies for their eventual lives as industrial workers. Indeed, infant care manuals of that era used industrial metaphors when describing feeding schedules: "make a machine of the little one, teach it to employ its various functions at fixed and convenient times" (The Youngest Member, 1889). The advice of the Women's Christian Temperance Union was equally urgent: in order to prevent alcoholism and drug addiction, mothers should not give in when infants cried for food (Wood-Allen, 1896).

For these compelling reasons, women adhered to feeding schedules so strictly that their complaints of not-enough-milk were probably valid. Feeding a newborn according to an every-four-hour, daytime-only schedule ensured a diminished milk supply and the need for artificial food. Although feeding schedules were not the sole reason for babies' consumption of cows' milk in the 1890s, mothers' complaints of inadequate milk invited doctors' involvement, and the medicalization of infant feeding would have profound consequences.

By the 1930s—after the dairy industry had cleaned up their filthy and spoiled product—a new generation of pediatricians who had never seen babies die for want of mothers' milk dismissed the importance of human milk to an infant's health, contrary to their predecessors. As one young St. Louis physician argued in 1931, "many uncontrollable factors enter in breast feeding." He urged mothers to rely on formula to "produce consistently normal growth and development" in their babies (Are Infant Feeding Methods Changing, 1931). Another typical doctor warned about human milk in 1934, "The fact that the fluid comes from the maternal mammary gland does not make it good. It may be nothing but water" (Tow, 1934). Today, the cultural message persists that while formula is steadfast and consistent, human milk is only randomly reliable. We face more than 140 years of culturally engrained belief that lactation is a uniquely unreliable body function, and that breasts are notoriously fickle body parts.

It Takes a Village

MOTHER'S MILK FOR MOTHER'S BABE
COW'S MILK FOR CALVES
(God's Plan)

The Long
vs.
The Short Haul

70 percent of city babies get their food through a tube 60 miles long.

It takes about 36 hours—often 42 hours—for the milk to run from the cow end of the tube to the baby end of the tube.

This tube is open in many places and baby's food is frequently polluted. It is often wrongly kept in overheated places.

Then there may be a diseased cow at the country end of the tube.

And Yet Some People Wonder Why So Many Babies Die!

On the other hand the mother-fed baby gets its milk fresh, pure and healthful—no germs can get into it.

To Lessen Baby Deaths Let Us Have More Mother-Fed Babies.

You can't improve on God's plan.

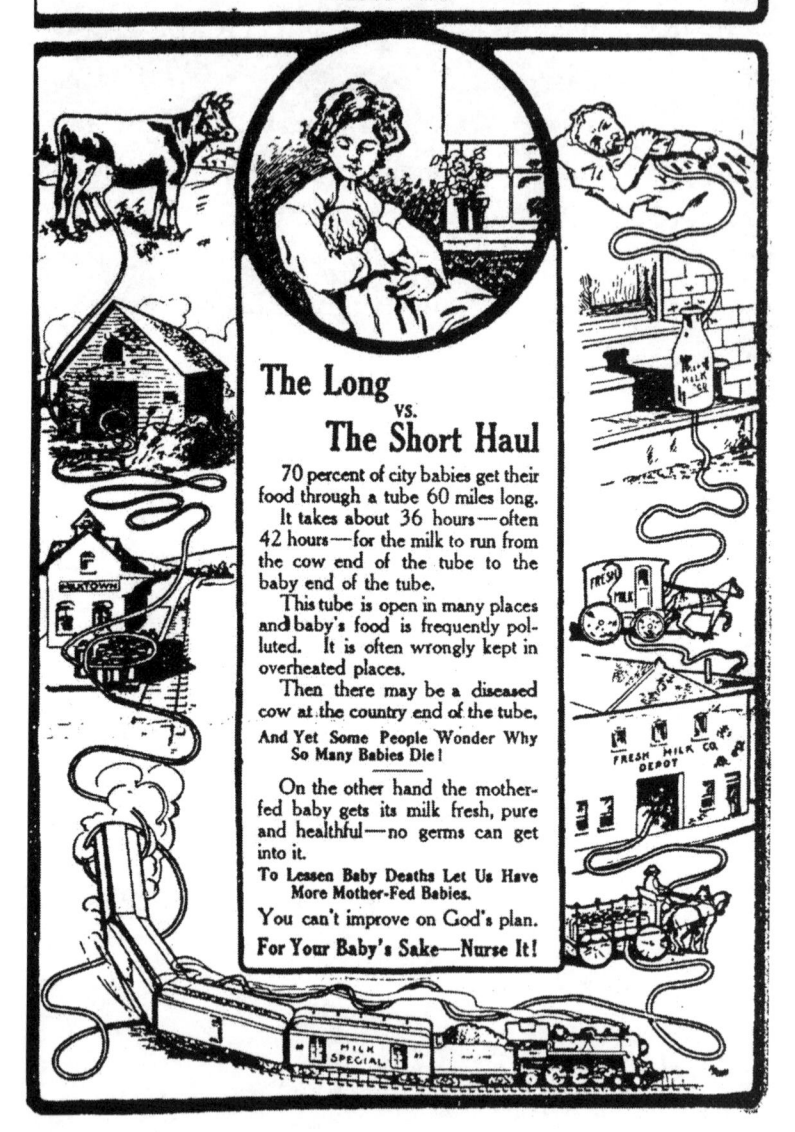

For Your Baby's Sake—Nurse It!

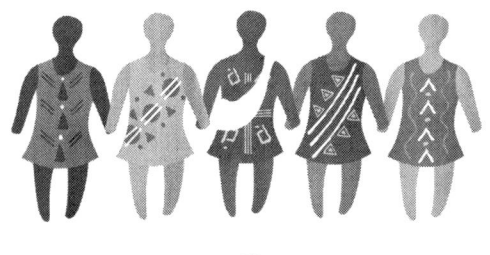

2

Eliminating Inequalities in Gender, Race, and Ethnicity

The Welfare State and the Breastfeeding Worker

Amanda Barnes Cook

What is the role of the state in accommodating breastfeeding workers? Scholars of welfare states have long discussed the different manner in which states provide for maternity leave, childcare provision, and other matters of policy related to balancing work and family, but they have not interrogated the way in which breastfeeding is (or is not) facilitated in the workplace (Esping-Anderson, 2002). Feminists and theorists of the welfare state alike argue that gender equity requires that workplaces are not hostile to women and that women have access to paid work (Orloff,

1993). Since 90% of women will become mothers in the course of their working lives (Williams, 2001), this means that the specific demands of motherhood, including and I argue especially, breastfeeding, must be facilitated by workplaces if we are to achieve gender equity. Thus, successful breastfeeding outcomes must be pursued in conjunction with gender equity in the feminist formulation of a new welfare state ideal.

Mothers who work outside the home are less likely to breastfeed. Laura Duberstein Lindberg (1996) finds that women were "more likely to stop breastfeeding if they were at work than if they were not employed" and that there is an "increased likelihood that women would stop breastfeeding in the 3-month interval marking their entrance to employment" (p. 248). State policies to help breastfeeding workers can come in a variety of packages: maternity leaves that are long enough to allow women to finish breastfeeding before they return to work, statutory establishment of the right of breastfeeding workers to breaks and to a space in which to pump at work, subsidies for on-site childcare, or tax benefits for the rental or purchase of breast pumps, for example.

In order to probe this issue, I look at the policies and breastfeeding outcomes in five countries: two liberal welfare states (the United States and the United Kingdom), one conservative welfare state (Germany), and two social democratic welfare states (Sweden and Norway). This case selection is chosen because it allows analysis of states with a wide variety of breastfeeding outcomes (ranging from the

UK, in which 7% of women are exclusively breastfeeding at four months, to Sweden, in which 61% of women are exclusively breastfeeding at four months), and will allow examination of difference between welfare-state regime types. In liberal regimes, mothers and families are left to reconcile the competing demands of care and work on an individual basis and usually within the private market. Conservative regimes, on the other hand, support mothers and families in the care of children through policies, such as lengthy maternity leave (often greater than a year), but do not support gender equality and women's ability to remain in the paid workforce. Social democratic regimes support mothers and families in the care of children through gender egalitarian policies, leave for mothers and fathers, and provision for part-time work for parents of young children, allowing women to "pursue motherhood within the work contract" (Ellingsaeter & Ronsen, 1996).

State Method to Accommodate and Promote Breastfeeding

I argue that state methods to accommodate and promote breastfeeding workers can be divided into three main categories: protective negative provisions, enabling positive provisions, and attempts to change cultural norms. **Protective negative provisions** are those that defend breastfeeding workers from discrimination or penalty for breastfeeding-related activities. **Enabling positive provisions** are those regulations that make it possible, in practice, for working mothers to choose to breastfeed without incurring undue costs. **Attempts to change cultural norms** are not generally aimed specifically at breastfeeding workers, but are projects at the state level that intend to render society more hospitable for those who choose to breastfeed—including working mothers. I postulate that these different types of accommodations may vary according to welfare state regime type, with liberal regimes offering mostly protective negative provisions, social democratic regimes offering both protective negative and enabling positive provisions, and conservative regimes falling in between and offering only those provisions that support traditional family structures.

In the cases considered, social democratic regimes have much higher breastfeeding durations than the other two regimes, with the liberal regimes falling on the lower end of the spectrum (Figure 1). The wide range of breastfeeding outcomes is indicative of the extent to which external factors influence breastfeeding initiation and duration. There is a 55 percentage point difference in breastfeeding rate at 6 months between Norway and the U.K. in 2005. While these outcomes are certainly not entirely explained by social policy (since other factors like culture and personal preference play a role), social policy is the place to begin to look for change since it is the only factor states can manipulate while leaving women in the ultimate position to make their own infant feeding choices.

I find that liberal welfare states leave it to individual women to navigate breastfeeding and work, providing protective negative provisions but few enabling positive

Eliminating Inequalities in Gender, Race, and Ethnicity

provisions for breastfeeding workers. Even the Affordable Care Act (ACA) in the U.S., though a step in the right direction, does not protect most women, does not allow for direct feeding of the infant, and only offers unpaid breaks. From the perspective of a mother returning to work a few short weeks after giving birth, this is nowhere near enough to accommodate a long-term breastfeeding relationship.

Breastfeeding Prevalence by Age, 2005*

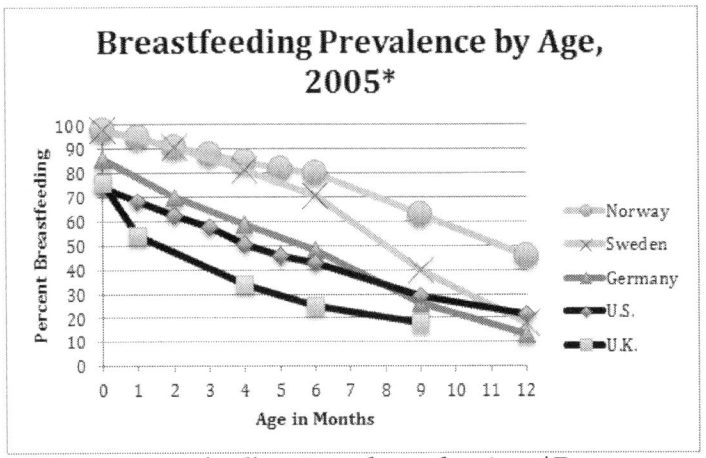

Figure 1. Breastfeeding Prevalence by Age *For comparative purposes with limited data collection, data presented is from 2005 for the US, UK, and Sweden; 2006-2007 for Norway; 1997 for Germany. *Sources: U.S. C.D.C.; U.K. N.H.S.; Norway Helsedirektoratet; Sweden Sveriges Officiella Statistik; Germany Kersting and Dulon.*

Conservative welfare states traditionally have offered both protective negative and enabling positive provisions for breastfeeding workers, but with less of an emphasis on allowing women to return to the workforce. Germany's breastfeeding rates fall in the middle. Germany's change to a more social democratic-style family policy may lead to a marked increase in breastfeeding rates over the next few years. It will be an interesting case to watch, and might shed insight on the effects of these programs in non-Scandinavian contexts. Social democratic welfare states actively pursue both gender equality and breastfeeding success through both protective negative and enabling positive provisions for breastfeeding workers, and also experience much higher rates of breastfeeding throughout the first year of life than the other regime types. Norway, especially, has an exceptionally high rate of breastfeeding at 12 months (46%).

To give mothers real choice about whether to breastfeed, I argue that the state has a role in designing institutions to facilitate breastfeeding workers. These case studies suggest that mothers are better able to achieve longer breastfeeding duration if states offer both negative protective provisions and positive enabling provisions to support breastfeeding workers, including paid maternity leave, work breaks in which to pump or nurse, and the right to part-time work for parents of young children. Moreover, to achieve both gender equality and successful breastfeeding outcomes, we need to pursue policy that allows women to take longer maternity leave at high replacement rates, during which time they can establish and enjoy the beginning or entirety of their breastfeeding relationship, followed by protections for breastfeeding mothers needing to pump on the job.

Father-only leave time is excellent from the perspective of gender equality, but it does not make sense to try to split leave time equally between parents, since fathers can't breastfeed and maternity leave is important for breastfeeding dyads. A system like Sweden's, where a mother can choose to stay home for 12 months, and then the father can stay home for an additional 4 months, is a reasonable solution: the mother is able to complete the most intense period of the breastfeeding relationship while on leave, and the father is able to split care and work when the child is a bit older. This minimizes the pumping burden on the mother, allows for successful breastfeeding outcomes, and an equitable split of caretaking work. This system also offers parents the most choice. It does not discriminate or shame mothers who do not breastfeed, while facilitating breastfeeding for those who choose to. It helps maintain high female labor force participation. It helps breastfeeding mothers, formula-feeding mothers, fathers, and children alike, and should garner broad support.

Breastfeeding Equity: Summary of a Concept Analysis

Ginny Combs

Breastfeeding as the optimal nutrition and biological norm for infants has been well established. Breastfeeding is a foundation of public health and must be seen as an essential link in the health continuum (Labbok & Nakaji, 2010). Although breastfeeding duration rates in the United States have shown small increases, the data suggested that we

It Takes a Village

have significant progress to make in overall duration rates and quality of breastfeeding supports for all women (CDC, 2012). This awareness of "all women" highlights a dimension of equity. *The Surgeon General's Call to Action to Support Breastfeeding* (2011) stressed that mothers face overwhelming challenges and significant disparities with the ability to breastfeed. The report goes on to appeal for the reduction of inequities in the quality of breastfeeding care mothers and infants receive. The intent of this analysis is to examine the concept of breastfeeding equity to develop greater insight for health care professionals as they examine their roles, assumptions, and overall views of breastfeeding. The theory of transformative learning proposed that it is only through critical reflection on meaning schemes, perspectives, propositions, beliefs, and assumptions that we can have greater insight (Mezirow & Associates, 1990).

Currently, most of the advocacy work for improving breastfeeding outcomes appears to emphasize the health benefits, techniques of feeding, and breastfeeding as a choice. However, there is a lack of comprehending the macro view of the breastfeeding experience. Moreover, breastfeeding in reality may not be a self-contained choice but rather, an institutional, social, and cultural construct with deeply ingrained barriers for women who want to breastfeed (Kukla, 2006). The CDC (2012) demonstrated the breastfeeding disparity for women in the United States to realize their breastfeeding goals. Women from ethnic minority groups and those from challenged socioeconomic groups have overall decreased breastfeeding rates. Cattaneo (2012) argued that without the use of an equity lens, advocacy for breastfeeding may be creating inequities. Labbok, Hall Smith, and Taylor (2008) insisted that breastfeeding be seen as a human reproductive right and that presently, the ability to act on this right is not a realistic choice for many women.

Definition

Equity as it relates to health care, human rights, health disparities, and social justice has been defined, explored, and refined over many years. Margaret Whitehead (1985), in her classic paper on equity, described a working definition as "Equity is therefore concerned with creating equal opportunities for health and with bringing health differential down to the lowest level possible" (p.7). Braveman (2006) expanded on the work of Whitehead and discussed equity in health as removing inequities for groups of people who are socially, economically, culturally, and racially disadvantaged. Maxwell (1992) proposed the use of specific questions to determine if services are equitable and recommended asking "Is this patient or group of patients being fairly treated relative to others?" (p.171).

Breastfeeding equity can be realized as the experience of fair opportunity by all women to actualize their breastfeeding goals regardless of variables, place, or time. For true breastfeeding equity to be present, the woman-infant dyad can enter the circle from any vantage point on the scale of life experience, and will have breastfeeding support, promotion, and protection with removal of barriers for those ideals (see Appendix for diagram). A woman can enter the circle from any direction and will have equal opportunities for equity, which is in opposition with the lived breastfeeding experience today for many women.

In her article on Inequalities and Inequities in Breastfeeding, Cattaneo (2012) laid out a foundation for understanding multiple dimensions of breastfeeding equity. For breastfeeding support, the author cited the importance of The Baby-Friendly Hospital Initiative, professional support, trained peer support, mother-to-mother support, and lay-person support, such as fathers and other relatives. According to Cattaneo, this will only promote breastfeeding equity if it is actively provided to disadvantaged women and communities. Breastfeeding equity can also be defined by promoting breastfeeding in communities of color and focusing on those communities with noted health disparities and low breastfeeding rates.

Attributes

Breastfeeding advocacy can be redesigned to represent the lived experience for breastfeeding by focusing on women of different colors and shapes breastfeeding in a variety of situations (Kukla, 2006). Seeing all types of women breastfeeding within promotional media would be an attribute of breastfeeding equity. It is crucial to take a step back and examine many of the current breastfeeding advocacy messages which present a particular view about the ease and appropriateness of breastfeeding and yet, the disconnect between what is recommended and what is experienced can be profound for women (Kukla, 2006). Breastfeeding equity can be seen visibly in the wide distribution of breastfeeding materials that encompass the whole of the breastfeeding experience for women. Critical to the area of promotion is the knowledge that for disadvantaged mothers, the risk of getting an incomplete or wrong message may reduce equity (Cattaneo, 2012). Additionally, another potential attribute of breastfeeding equity may the normalization of breastfeeding in elementary, middle, and high school education.

To grasp how the United States might value breastfeeding equity, one must realize that up until the 2010 "reasonable break time" provision of the Patient Protection and Affordable Care Act, women had no protection or right to breastfeed at work (Murtagh & Moulton, 2011). As it stands, the current legislation leaves out many working mothers and is only a beginning in the laws needed for breastfeeding equity to be realized. As Labbok et al. (2008) eloquently reasoned, "It is important to re-orient the paradigm from the current view that breastfeeding is a 'lifestyle' choice, to a paradigm that views breastfeeding as a reproductive health, rights, and social justice issue so as to ensure the social, economic, and political conditions necessary to promote success" (p. 2). Breastfeeding equity can only happen with a full alignment of organizational, policy, community, and individual/family changes and strategies (Labbok et al., 2008), as well as viewing breastfeeding as a society-shared responsibility (McKinley & Hyde, 2004).

Consequences

Bartek and Reinhold (2010) stressed the significance of "suboptimal" breastfeeding related to the United States population and economy. Their data suggested that 13 billion dollars per year, and 911 deaths, could be prevented as a result of 90% of families in the United States breastfeeding for six months. The consequences of breastfeeding equity could therefore be the opposite of suboptimal breastfeeding in terms of cost savings and infant mortality.

Empirical Referents

How would one know the existence of breastfeeding equity? Braveman (2006) submitted that health equity be measured by the comparison of an indicator of health in one or more disadvantaged groups with the same indicator in a more advantaged group. Breastfeeding equity referents could be the statistical data regarding breastfeeding rates and duration among diverse populations of women along with the detailed variables of support, protection, and promotion of breastfeeding within each group.

Conclusion

The United States Surgeon General, in *The Call to Action to Support Breastfeeding* (2011), provides a powerful appeal for breastfeeding when she asserted "Rarely are we given the chance to make such a profound and lasting difference in the lives of so many." Comprehending breastfeeding equity provides a framework for understanding how to intervene and partner with mothers and families to provide optimal breastfeeding support, promotion and protection.

Milk and Motherhood: Breastfeeding and "Good Motherhood" Among African American Women in the South

Taylor Livingston

In May 2012 the cover of *Time* magazine showed a White woman breastfeeding a toddler with the caption: "Are you Mom Enough?" implying that a complete mother is one who breastfeeds. The *Time* cover reflects the current trend in public health to portray breastfeeding as a marker of "good motherhood." However, this conceptualization has not been uniformly embraced, particularly among African American women, who continue to have substantially lower breastfeeding rates than their White and Latina counterparts (Centers for Disease Control and Prevention, 2011).

The public health literature, which considers African American women's breastfeeding rates as a problem, abounds on the possible explanations for low breastfeeding rates among African American women. Yet, anthropology has been silent on the topic. Indeed, anthropologists have not examined breastfeeding among African American women, nor African American motherhood. My project attempts to fill in this gap by examining what it means to be a "good African American mother," and who or what influences the practices that this ideology incorporates. Further, the concern about African American mothers is especially relevant in the South, where the historical memory of the wet-nursing practices of slavery, the raping of slave women, and other abuses of Black women's bodies, the over-sexualization of Black women's bodies, and racist views of Black motherhood, continues to affect the motherhood experiences today. Durham, North Carolina lies within this Southern ethnographic milieu and adds its own unique context.

Durham has a rich African American history. The city was home to Hayti, an African American settlement that flourished from 1868 to 1940, and also one of the nation's strongest economic African American districts known as "Black Wall Street" (Anderson, 2011.) Durham also has a unique relationship with breastfeeding and motherhood. As mentioned above, Durham is a site of multiple research projects on breastfeeding, possibly because its breastfeeding rates for African American women at initiation, six months, and one year marks are comparable to those for African Americans in the U.S. (Labbok & Taylor, 2010). Durham also has an interesting relationship with African Americans and motherhood, as non-consensual sterilizations were performed on Black women in North Carolina until 1972.

Using this history as my foundation, and the theoretical notions of "the embodiment of history" (Fassin, 2007), Black feminist theory on the abuses of Black women's bodies (Collins, 2004; Roberts, 1997), and "authoritative knowledge" (Jordan, 1993; Martin, 1987) as my guides, I undertake ethnographic research employing surveys, semi-structured interviews, focus groups, and generational interviews to explore possible explanations for African American women's approaches to infant feeding. Ultimately, I explore how breastfeeding fits into larger historically situated notions of what it means to be a "good African American mother" in the U.S., especially the U.S. South. As such, my project asks the following research questions:

1. What does it mean to be a "good mother" for African American women in the U.S. South? Are there diverse meanings of "good motherhood" among African women and do these vary by social location?

2. How do Southern African American women's conceptualizations of "good motherhood" relate to breastfeeding?

3. Which actors (e.g., public health campaigns, health care professionals, family, peer networks, institutional memberships) are influential in shaping what African American women consider to be appropriate practices for achieving "good mothering"?

4. To what extent have historical events influenced African American mothers' thoughts, practices, and feelings about motherhood and breastfeeding?

In asking these questions, my goal is to reorient the focus adopted by public health researchers who contend that there are socioeconomic and support barriers that prevent African American women from breastfeeding. This research assumes that if these barriers were removed, the rates of breastfeeding among African American women would increase. It is indeed possible that these dynamics play some role in shaping a woman's decision to breastfeed. Yet, my project brings insights from diverse literatures in feminism, medical anthropology, and cultural anthropology to allow us to go beyond a consideration of material constraints, and to instead consider the role that meanings of motherhood play in infant feeding decisions and practices.

Method

The sample population for this research project is comprised of pregnant, exclusively breastfeeding, breastfeeding and formula-feeding, or exclusively formula-feeding women who identify as African American, or identify as having African American heritage in Durham, NC. Women will be recruited at entry into prenatal care and screened for eligibility criteria. A sample of 60 women will be selected based on a representative sample of the various socioeconomic statuses, educational backgrounds, marital statuses, and ages of the women in this project. Women will complete a survey providing information about their educational background, age, marital status, employment status, views of breastfeeding, infant feeding intentions (formula-feeding, breastfeeding, or both), and practices they think "good mothers" perform. To answer my question regarding historical abuses of Black women's bodies, racist views of Black motherhood, and the legacy of the over-sexualization of

Black women's bodies, I will conduct focus groups and generational interviews with the women enrolled in this study and their matrilineal kin.

Guiding Arguments

My expectations for what my data will show are broad and serve as a general and flexible guide in my project. Because we know so little about African American women's views on motherhood in anthropology, asserting strict, literature-informed hypotheses is not possible. Thus, as an alternative, I offer general and open expectations or arguments, informed by specific social theories of race and gender; history and race; and gender and medicalization.

At the broadest level, I am arguing that African American women's meanings and practices of motherhood will be shaped by their social connections and experience, past and present. Because Southern African American women's regional and socio-historical experiences are not "the norm" in the U.S., I expect that African American women's views on mothering will not fully reflect conventions of motherhood at a national level previously documented by anthropologists, feminist scholars, and public health researchers. This includes the convention of breastfeeding as a feature of "good mothering" in the 21st century.

I am arguing that, instead of the national conventions and predominant discourses about mothering, a variety and hybrid of non-biomedical, non-public health "authoritative knowledges"(Jordan, 1993; Martin, 1987), drawn directly from African American women's social networks and experiences, will inform their views on mothering and infant feeding. These experiences include, but may not be limited to, enduring histories. That is, past (antebellum through mid-20th century) approaches to Southern African American women's bodies in biomedicine, by the state, and on plantations may also inform how African American women conceive of what is appropriate and preferable mothering and infant feeding.

As with the long range impact of the famous Tuskegee study on Black males' acceptance of biomedical perspectives, information about these histories circulates across generations and time, and may be influential in how Black women approach the use of their bodies for infant care. Thus, African American women's meanings of motherhood, formed out of their social location and experience, are critical to understanding their infant care decisions. Importantly, understanding such meanings should provide broader insights into what public health officials consider to be the conundrum of African American women's relatively low breastfeeding rates.

Conclusion

By undertaking this dissertation research, I show what anthropological investigations can do by "talking back" (Hooks, 1987) to public health discourses and government agencies that urge women to breastfeed exclusively for six months, and continue breastfeeding while supplementing with solid foods for one year or more, but do not consider why this discourse has not been received by all women, and why certain women may not be able to do so. Additionally, this research will help increase local and national breastfeeding rates by providing information on possible reasons why women may not breastfeed. This information is valuable for political reasons, as large-scale structural reform policies could help overcome these issues, and as a matter of national concern as babies who are not breastfed have more doctors' visits and hospitalizations. Further, the findings of this research will be reported back to La Leche League, WIC clinics, and lactation consultants, the largest support providers of lactation support, in order to help to understand why public health discourses promoting breastfeeding are not adhered to by all women. Further, a report of my research findings will be sent to the Department of Health and Human Services Office on Women and the Center, the Center for Disease Control, the North Carolina Department of Health Services, and the North Carolina Breastfeeding Coalition.

It Takes a Village

Undoing Institutional Racism in Perinatal Support Organizations: First Steps for Eliminating Racial Inequity in Breastfeeding Support

Cynthia Good Mojab and Emily Healy

Background

The United States is making progress nationally in breastfeeding initiation and duration (Centers for Disease Control and Prevention 2012): more than three out of four mothers (76.9%) in the United States start out breastfeeding, and 47% of U.S. babies are breastfed for at least 6 months, but only 16% are exclusively breastfed. However, breastfeeding rates for Black infants are about 50% lower than those for White infants at birth, six months, and 12 months—even when controlling for the family's income or education levels (Centers for Disease Control and Prevention, 2012; U.S. Department of Health and Human Services, 2011).

Even in developed countries, such as the U.S., not breastfeeding is associated with increased risk of infant mortality and morbidity, including infectious diseases, childhood obesity, type 1 and 2 diabetes, leukemia, and Sudden Infant Death Syndrome. It is also associated with increased health risks for mothers, including ovarian cancer, premenopausal breast cancer, myocardial infarction, retained gestational weight gain, type 2 diabetes, and metabolic syndrome (Stuebe, 2009). Lower initiation and duration rates of breastfeeding serve as a vehicle for poorer health outcomes for Black infants and their mothers. African American infants are 2.4 times more likely than White infants to die in their first year of life (Collins & David, 2009).

Institutional Racism in White Perinatal Support Organizations

Closing the racial gap in breastfeeding rates is required to eliminate racial inequities in maternal-infant health. One way to reduce racial inequities in breastfeeding initiation and duration is to increase the access of mothers of color to peer and professional breastfeeding support. Peer and professional breastfeeding support has been proven to improve breastfeeding rates (e.g., Chapman et al., 2010; Rishel & Sweeney, 2005). However, mainstream mother-to-mother breastfeeding support organizations, and other mainstream perinatal organizations that serve breastfeeding mothers in the U.S., tend to be disproportionately White-led institutions that disproportionately serve White mothers (Good Mojab, 2013; Seals Allers, 2012a, 2012b). While these organizations contribute significantly to the health and development of the mostly White mothers and infants whom they serve well, they are not adequately meeting the needs of communities of color.

The disproportionate Whiteness of mainstream organizations that provide breastfeeding support in the U.S. is a manifestation of institutional racism in breastfeeding support. Institutional racism has been defined as a "systemic and structural problem that creates [an] institution-

It Takes a Village

al mono-culture that makes it difficult for People of Color, immigrants, and refugees to access and receive services in culturally sensitive and appropriate ways" (Crossroads Anti-Racism Organizing and Training, 2011). According to Jones (2000), institutional racism is:

> differential access to the goods, services, and opportunities of society by race. Institutionalized racism is normative, sometimes legalized, and often manifests as inherited disadvantage. It is structural, having been codified in our institutions of custom, practice, and law, so there need not be an identifiable perpetrator. Indeed, institutionalized racism is often evident as inaction in the face of need.

Clearly, increasing access of mothers of color to peer and professional breastfeeding support requires the dismantling of institutional racism in perinatal support organizations.

Beginning Anti-Racism Work in White Perinatal Support Organizations

The authors are familiar with anti-racism work engaged in by several predominantly White perinatal support organizations that provide midwifery, doula, and breastfeeding services. Our observation and experience is that the process of dismantling institutional racism is very difficult, especially in its beginning stages. While the anti-racism expertise of a largely White organization's members may vary from non-existent to substantial, most members are novices. Common first steps of anti-racism work include forming an anti-racism committee, self-education within the committee, the committee providing education to the larger organization, the committee beginning to collaborate with colleagues and organizations of color outside of the organization, the committee proposing a plan of action, and the organization taking initial action (e.g., publishing an inclusivity statement).

Those who are committed to dismantling institutional racism within the organization may feel hope and excitement about moving toward serving communities of color more equitably. That enthusiasm is soon tempered by the encountering of common barriers in the beginning of antiracism work, such as resistance within the organization to training, resistance within the organization to needed change, and the departure of members committed to anti-racism work due to disillusionment with the organization's resistance. In the beginning stages, anti-racism committee members, and other members of the organization, may not realize the long-term nature of the work, have sufficient knowledge and tools to move the work forward, nor have sufficient commitment from the organization's leadership to be able to take effective and substantial action.

Well-meaning Whites working in the field of perinatal support are commonly first drawn to engage in steps that can be taken relatively quickly and easily, such as diversifying images of mothers and babies in publications, changing service locations, and engaging in outreach to communities

It Takes a Village

of color. While these may be legitimate steps, they are insufficient. "In-reach" is much more important than outreach. The structures of the organization that perpetuate racism must be dismantled and rebuilt based on a systemic analysis of the nature of institutional racism within the organization. It is not enough for an organization to perceive itself as "welcoming" of families of color. The organization must change policies and procedures so that its services actually meet the needs of the *entire* community and its power holders, and service providers are representative of the *entire* community that it serves.

Predominantly White perinatal support organizations can gain ideas, hope, and accountability by modeling and supporting the work of organizations that strive to eliminate racial inequity in perinatal support services and outcomes, such as The Birth Place in Winter Garden, Florida; the International Center for Traditional Childbearing in Portland, Oregon; Reaching Our Sisters Everywhere (ROSE) in Lithonia, Georgia; Uzazi Village in Kansas City, Missouri; and Open Arms Perinatal Services in Seattle, Washington. White-led perinatal support organizations that persevere through the inevitable internal resistance to dismantling institutional racism will eventually make progress. More experienced White-led perinatal support organizations that are in various stages of dismantling institutional racism can also serve as role models to beginners of what to do—and not to do—such as Bastyr University's Department of Midwifery (Yglesia, 2012) and the United States Breastfeeding Coalition (USBC, 2011).

Call to Action

In spite of the challenges that dismantling institutional racism poses, racial inequities in breastfeeding rates and access to breastfeeding support cannot be eliminated without it. Perinatal organizations that want to become part of the solution must engage in many different steps that will help them create more just practices, policies, and structures (Crossroads Anti-racism Organizing and Training, 2007; Seattle Human Services Coalition, 2005). Such steps include:

Providing anti-racism training to all members of the organization, starting with those in positions of power (e.g., members of the Board of Directors, department heads, committee chairs).

- Requesting input from, utilizing the input of, and better supporting people of color who are already working within or served by the organization.

- Developing accountability to, collaborating with, and supporting the work of organizations of color that are already providing services to communities of color.

- Reconstructing policies, procedures, and structures in a manner that measurably removes barriers to access to breastfeeding support, education, credentialing, and other services provided by the organization to mothers and service providers of color, for example, by:

- Establishing a baseline of the current status of breastfeeding support, education, credentialing, and other services provided by the organization to mothers and service providers of color.

- Formally assessing on an annual basis the degree and nature of institutional racism within the organization.

- Incorporating into the organization's bylaws and strategic plans a mandate for socially representative racial and ethnic diversification of the Board of Directors and service providers.

- Recreating organizational statements (e.g., mission, vision) that explicitly express a commitment to anti-racism.

- Providing resources and mandatory training on an annual basis to all power holders and service providers on how to increase their cultural competence and counter institutional racism in their areas of responsibility.

- Redesigning or changing the selection of materials produced or used by the organization so as to ensure socially representative diversity and cultural competence of their content.

Conclusion

Continued racial inequities in breastfeeding support, breastfeeding rates, and maternal-infant health outcomes are unacceptable. All perinatal support organizations and service providers can and must find a way to do their part to dismantle institutional racism. While this work is difficult, it is essential to fulfilling the implicitly and explicitly inclusive visions and missions of perinatal support organizations in an increasingly diverse world. Fortunately, many resources and role models are available to individuals and organizations that are just beginning their anti-racism journey. There is strength in numbers: the more perinatal support organizations and service providers add their voices and actions to the work of dismantling institutional racism, the sooner we will develop the critical mass needed to fully eliminate the breastfeeding gap created by racism.

Mothers and Others: An Intervention with Promise for Improving Breastfeeding Outcomes among African American Women

Heather Wasser, Cynthia Bulik, Myles Faith, Barbara Goldman, Eric Hodges, Eliana Perrin, Chirayath Suchindran, Amanda Thompson, and Margaret Bentley

To maximize health benefits for both mother and child, the American Academy of Pediatrics (AAP), and the World Health Organization (WHO) encourage women to breastfeed exclusively for the first six months, and to continue breastfeeding, alongside the introduction of complementary foods, for the infant's first year of life or longer (Eidelman, 2012; Horta & Victora, 2013a, 2013b). In the United States, the majority of women giving birth choose to breastfeed (81.9% in 2011), but much smaller proportions are meeting recommendations for exclusivity or continued breastfeeding, and rates are particularly low for African American women (Bentley, Gavin, Black, & Teti, 1999; Center for Disease Control and Prevention, 2007). National rates by race show that just 14.4%, 13.4%, and 8.2% of White, Hispanic, and African American women, respectively, are exclusively breastfeeding until 6 months, and 23.6%, 24.7%, and 12.9% of White, Hispanic and African American women, respectively, are still breastfeeding at one year (Center for Disease Control and Prevention, 2007). The purpose of this paper is to describe a promising obesity prevention intervention, *Mothers and Others*, which includes secondary outcomes aimed at improving breastfeeding rates among African American women.

Study Aims

The primary aim of *Mothers and Others* is to conduct a randomized controlled trial (NCT01938118) among 468 African American pregnant women, their families, and their child caregivers to test the efficacy of a multi-component, tailored intervention versus an attention control (child safety) to promote healthy weight gain patterns during infancy

(Main Outcomes). We hypothesize that infants of families in the intervention versus attention control group will display significantly healthier growth outcomes, including: 1) a lower mean weight-for-length z-score (WLZ) at 18 months; 2) a smaller change in mean WLZ between 0-18 months; and, 3) a lower likelihood of overweight (WLZ ≥ 95th percentile) at 18 months.

A secondary aim of *Mothers and Others* is to determine if the intervention is successful in increasing targeted health behaviors, including breastfeeding outcomes, and test whether these behaviors are predictive of healthy weight gain patterns. We hypothesize that a higher proportion of women in the intervention versus attention control group will initiate breastfeeding, will be exclusively breastfeeding at 3 and 6 months, and will continue to breastfeed until 12 months. A final aim of *Mothers and Others* is to use mediation analyses to ascertain whether the targeted health behaviors were achieved through the modifiable factors/behavioral determinants underpinning the intervention.

We hypothesize that the breastfeeding outcomes will be partially mediated by one or more of the following behavioral determinants: 1) more positive breastfeeding attitudes; 2) higher levels of breastfeeding self-efficacy; 3) higher levels of social support; 4) higher responsive feeding style scores; 5) improved accuracy in perceiving infant and toddler weight status; and 6) diminished perceptions of infant fussiness.

Recruitment and Enrollment

We will draw our study population from women seeking prenatal care through obstetric and gynecologic clinics serving two major hospitals in central North Carolina. Individuals eligible to participate in the study will include African American women with a singleton pregnancy, English-speaking, and <28 weeks pregnant. Exclusion criteria will include prematurity (gestation <36 weeks); birth weight <2500 grams; newborn nursery, NICU, or maternity stay > 7 days; or diagnosis of a congenital anomaly or other condition that significantly affects feeding (e.g., Down's syndrome, cleft lip, or palate). The sequence generation process will be based on a random number table that incorporates stratification by hospital and maternal age. Participants will be randomized to study group after giving informed consent and completing the baseline survey. Study staff randomizing participants will use a web-based allocation that blinds group allocation.

Intervention Description

Both study arms will begin during the second trimester of pregnancy and continue into the second year of life. Primary modes of delivery include face-to-face counseling through home visits, health newsletters, and ~160 cue-based text messages. Study components for the intervention group have been designed to create more positive breastfeeding attitudes, higher levels of breastfeeding self-efficacy, and greater social support for breastfeeding. The majority of home visits for the intervention group will be delivered by a local African American mother, who is also a Certified Lactation Counselor. These visits will occur at approximately 30 and 34 weeks gestation and 3, 6, 9, and 12 months postpartum.

Topics to be covered during the prenatal home visits include the benefits of breastfeeding, anticipatory guidance about infant behavior (cues, crying, and sleep), techniques for building a good milk supply (e.g., early skin-to-skin, minimal swaddling, cluster feeding), and strategies for mobilizing social support once the baby is born. Topics related to breastfeeding during the postpartum home visits include ongoing guidance about infant behavior, managing breastfeeding while returning to work or school, breastfeeding while introducing complementary foods, and weaning. Participants in the intervention group will also receive two home visits from an International Board Certified Lactation Consultant (IBCLC) shortly after returning home from the hospital and unlimited access to an IBCLC through phone calls and/or email up until 12 months postpartum.

Topics are reinforced through newsletters delivered between home visits and twice weekly text messages. Given the important role of interpersonal relationships on women's infant feeding practices, most notably the attitudes and opinions of fathers, grandmothers, and friends, women in the intervention group will also choose a study partner (Center for Disease Control and Prevention, 2014; DiGirolamo, Thompson, Martorell, Fein, & Grummer-Strawn, 2005; Meedya, Fahy, & Kable, 2010). Study partners will be encouraged to attend home visits and will also receive newsletters and text messages. The control group will receive home visits at approximately 30 and 34 weeks gestation and 3, 6, 9, and 12 months postpartum, as well as newsletters and text messages. Topics for the control group will be adapted for home use using the anticipatory guidance on child safety and injury prevention published in the *American Academy of Pediatrics' Bright Futures* (3rd Ed.) (*http://brightfutures.aap.org/*).

Data Collection

Data will be collected at baseline (28 weeks gestation), 36 weeks gestation, and 1, 3, 6, 9, 12, and 18 months postpartum. Infant birth weight and length will be abstracted from hospital records. Using standardized equipment, weight and length at subsequent time points will be measured in the home by trained study staff according to guidelines used in the existing NHANES survey. Infant dietary intake will be measured in two ways: an Infant Diet History (IDH) adapted after the IDH used in the Infant Feeding Practices II Study (Fein, Labiner-Wolfe, Shealy, Li, Chen, & Grummer-Strawn, 2008), and at 18 months, a series of three 24-hour dietary recalls (24-h DRs). Other relevant measures include the Infant Feeding Intentions Scale (Nommsen-Rivers & Dewey, 2009), which will be administered at baseline and 36 weeks pregnancy; breastfeeding attitudes of mothers and study partners, which will be assessed using the Iowa Infant Feeding Attitudes Scale (IIFAS) (De La Mora & Russell, 1999) administered at baseline and 36 weeks pregnancy; and the Breastfeeding Self-Efficacy Scale – Short Form (BSES-SF) (Dennis, 2003) administered to mothers at 1 month postpartum.

Conclusion

Mothers and Others is an innovative study designed to meet the unique needs of individual families by delivering anticipatory guidance on infant care, feeding, and growth through multiple channels and to multiple caregivers. If successful in achieving greater rates of breastfeeding initiation, exclusivity, and duration, *Mothers and Others* will have high public health relevance for future breastfeeding promotion efforts targeted to African American women and families.

Differences in Early Breastfeeding Experiences and Outcomes in Spanish versus English-Speaking Latinas from the Early Lactation Success Study Cohort of First-Time Mothers

Erin A. Wagner, Caroline J. Chantry, Kathryn G. Dewey, and Laurie A. Nommsen-Rivers

Recent census data show that more than half of the population growth in the United States from 2000-2010 can be attributed to an increase in the Hispanic population (Passel, Cohn, & Lopez, 2011), and that Hispanics represent over a quarter of the current U.S. infant population. Latinas in the United States have higher breastfeeding rates than non-Hispanic Whites of comparable economic or educational background (Singh, Kogan, & Dee, 2007). Paradoxically, however, they also have higher formula supplementation rates in the first two days postpartum compared with non-Hispanic Whites or Blacks (Centers for Disease Control and Prevention, 2007).

Many studies among U.S. Latinas have indicated that increased acculturation to the United States is associated with less optimal breastfeeding outcomes (Ahluwalia, D'Angelo, Morrow, & McDonald, 2012; Chapman & Perez-Escamilla, 2011; Guendelman & Siega-Riz, 2002; Singh et al., 2007). Immigrants from societies where breastfeeding is the norm may have more familiarity with and positive attitudes towards breastfeeding as compared to the United States, where general attitudes towards breastfeeding are ambivalent (Li, Rock, & Grummer-Strawn, 2007). However, little research has been done to elucidate specific factors that may explain why in the United States, acculturation is associated with less optimal breastfeeding outcomes in Latinas, particularly in women of Mexican American heritage.

The objective of this secondary analysis was to use data from Latina participants in the Early Lactation Success (ELS) study to explore possible reasons for the differences in breastfeeding outcomes by primary language (Spanish vs. English), used as a proxy for acculturation. We examined the following questions:

1. Are breastfeeding outcomes better for Spanish-speaking (presumably less-acculturated) compared to English-speaking (presumably more acculturated) Latinas in the ELS cohort?

2. Are there differences in breastfeeding attitudes, intentions, and support between Spanish- and English-speaking Latinas in the ELS cohort?

3. Do Spanish- and English-speaking Latinas report different problems and concerns with breastfeeding and different strategies for resolving them? Which strategies are associated with better breastfeeding outcomes at two months?

Method

The ELS study was a prospective cohort study completed at the University of California Davis Medical Center (UCMDC) in Sacramento, CA. The objective was to examine the barriers to establishing breastfeeding among first-time mothers of healthy, term infants. Between January 2006 and December 2007, the study enrolled 532 English- or Spanish-speaking expectant primiparae between 32 and 40 weeks gestation. Exclusion criteria included age <18 years and unable to obtain parental consent, living outside an 8-mile radius of the UCDMC, known contraindication to breastfeeding, or medical referral to UCDMC.

Participants who delivered at term and initiated breastfeeding (447) were followed until 60 days postpartum (or until breastfeeding terminated). Self-reported ethnicity and breastfeeding attitudes, self-efficacy (Dennis, 2006), intentions (Nommsen-Rivers, Cohen, Chantry, & Dewey, 2010), and concerns were assessed prenatally. In-person follow-up interviews were conducted within 24 hours of giving birth (Day 0), between 72 and 96 hours of giving birth (Day 3), and at 1 week postpartum (Day 7). Telephone interviews were completed at 2 weeks (Day 14), 1 month (Day 30) and 2 months (Day 60) postpartum. At each follow-up interview, feeding patterns were assessed, and mothers were asked to "please describe any problems or concerns you have had since our last interview or are currently having about feeding your baby, including breastfeeding problems, concerns, or discomforts" and, for each concern, how they attempted to resolve it and from whom they sought help.

Open text responses were grouped into major categories. Differences between Spanish and English-speaking Latina groups were determined using chi-square test.

Results

Contextual Differences and Outcomes

Among the 114 participants in the ELS cohort who reported Hispanic ethnicity (86% reported Mexican heritage) and who had breastfeeding outcome data, there were 52 whose primary language was Spanish, and 62 whose primary language was English. Spanish-speaking Latinas were significantly younger, much more likely to be born outside the U.S., have low income, and participate in WIC than English-speaking Latinas (Table 1). Almost all the English-speaking participants, but less than half of the Spanish-speaking participants, reported plans to go back to school or work outside of the home within the year.

Although Spanish-speaking and English-speaking Latinas were similar in prenatal breastfeeding intentions, breastfeeding self-efficacy, and in-hospital formula supplementation (Table 1), by 60 days postpartum English-speaking Latinas were almost three times more likely than Spanish-speakers to have stopped breastfeeding (31% vs. 11%, $p<0.01$, Figure 1). Spanish-speakers were more likely than English-speaking participants to report that their mother and sisters/close female relatives had breastfed their infants. Spanish-speaking Latinas were more likely to have the highest score on a composite measure of environmental support for breastfeeding (i.e., reporting that most/all family members are supportive of breastfeeding, reporting breastfeeding to be more convenient than bottle feeding, and not finding breastfeeding embarrassing, 67% vs. 34%, $p=0.003$).

Breastfeeding Concerns and Problems and Strategies for Overcoming Them

We previously characterized reported breastfeeding problems and concerns for the entire cohort and identified 50 distinct breastfeeding concerns that we consolidated into nine categories (manuscript in submission). Overall, there were few differences in reports of breastfeeding concerns between the Spanish and English-speaking Latinas. Spanish-speakers (vs. English-speakers) were less likely to report "infant feeding difficulty" as a prenatal concern (10% vs. 32%, $p<0.005$), and "uncertainty about own ability to breastfeed" at Day 0 (10% vs. 24%, $p=0.04$) and Day 14 (8% vs. 22%, $p=0.04$). Spanish-speakers were more likely to report "milk quantity concern" at Day 3 (47% vs. 28%, $p=0.04$), but not at other time points.

In categorizing the sources of help and the strategies that participants reported for resolving their breastfeeding concerns, we decided to first look specifically at strategies for resolving "infant feeding difficulty" and "milk quantity concern" at the Day 7 interview, because they were common concerns and had a strong relationship with breastfeeding outcomes in the larger cohort.

Fifty-one Latina participants reported a concern about "infant feeding difficulty," and 28 reported a milk quantity concern at the Day 7 interview. About a third of both English- and Spanish-speakers sought help for infant feeding difficulty from the UCDMC early lactation follow-up clinic; a quarter of Spanish-speakers sought help from a WIC lactation consultant, though this was not a common source of help for English-speakers; and over a quarter of English-speakers reported seeking help from no one (which was uncommon for Spanish-speakers). Other sources of help included a nurse, physician, or lactation consultant at the UCDMC hospital, family member, friend, or breastfeeding informational materials. For milk quantity concern at Day 7, a third of English-speakers and half of Spanish-speakers reported that they sought help from no one (the most common response); a third of English-speakers (but only 10% of Spanish-speakers) sought help from the UCDMC early lactation follow-up clinic.

The most common categories for strategies for resolving infant feeding difficulty at Day 7 were responses specifically mentioning feeding at the breast (includes references to positioning the baby, latch technique, frequent feeding, and feeding with a nipple shield), reported by approximately half of both English- and Spanish-speakers; a psychosocial approach (includes references to reassurance, keep trying, or resolving with time), reported by half of English- and a quarter of Spanish-speakers); and avoiding breastfeeding (includes references to feeding expressed breast milk rather than breastfeeding or using formula), reported by a quarter of both groups.

For those reporting milk quantity concern at Day 7, approximately half of both groups reported coping by avoiding breastfeeding, which was the most commonly reported strategy. Pumping was mentioned by about half of English-speakers but only a third of Spanish-speakers. Monitoring (i.e., monitoring the physical presence of milk, the baby's cues, or weight status) was reported by about 40% of both groups, and a psychosocial approach was mentioned by about a third of both groups.

Because of the small sample size, it was not possible to look at the relationship of particular strategies with breastfeeding outcomes stratified by primary language. However, when combining the two language groups, those who reported using a psychosocial strategy (either alone or in combination with another strategy) to address either an infant feeding difficulty or milk quantity concern at Day 7 had similarly high prevalence of continued breastfeeding at 60 days postpartum as those who did not report either concern, whereas those who did not report using a psychosocial strategy had lower prevalence of continued breastfeeding at 60 days ($p<0.05$, Figure 2).

Discussion

In Latinas from the ELS cohort, the gap in early breastfeeding outcomes between Spanish- and English-speakers does not appear to be explained by differences in prenatal breastfeeding intentions. It is possible that high breastfeeding self-efficacy and a supportive environment for breastfeeding (support of close family and friends and not perceiving breastfeeding to be embarrassing or inconvenient),

Eliminating Inequalities in Gender, Race, and Ethnicity

or less postpartum work or school obligations contribute to better breastfeeding outcomes in Spanish-speaking relative to English-speaking Latinas. This is consistent with results

Figure 1 - *Breastfeeding Outcomes at 60 Days Postpartum*

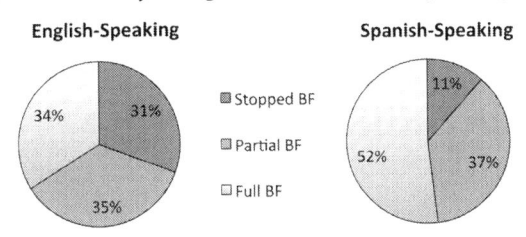

English-Speaking: 34% Stopped BF, 31% Partial BF, 35% Full BF

Spanish-Speaking: 11% Stopped BF, 37% Partial BF, 52% Full BF

Full breastfeeding defined as reporting having given no formula, other milk, or solids between Day 30 and Day 60 interview

Figure 2 - *Report of Psychosocial Strategy to Resolve Infant Feeding Difficulty (N=51) or Milk Quantity Concern (N=28) at Day 7 and Breastfeeding at 60 Days Postpartum*

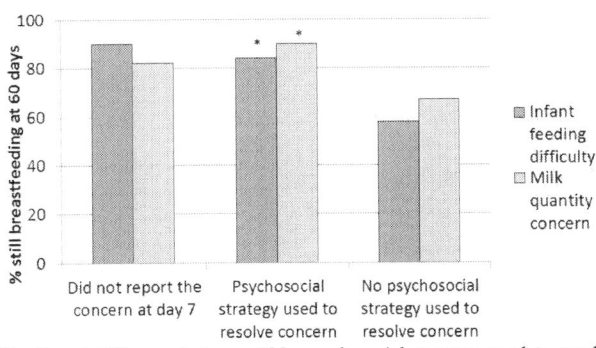

*Significant difference between "No psychosocial strategy used to resolve concern," $p<0.05$

from a study of Latina immigrants of predominantly Mexican origin living in California (survey completed in 1992-1993). Guendelman and Siega-Riz (2002) found that among participants living the longest in the U.S. (>15 years), 47% said that personal plans regarding work or school contributed to their decision to stop breastfeeding; this was not a common response, however, for those who were less acculturated.

The gap in early breastfeeding outcomes between Spanish- and English-speakers also does not seem to be explained by differences in types of breastfeeding problems or concerns experienced. However, data from our cohort suggest that psychosocial support—in concert with practical lactation support—may help Latina women to overcome their problems and concerns, and continue breastfeeding.

Acknowledgements

We would like to thank our study participants; staff at the UCDMC; University of California, Davis students and staff who contributed to this study; and Jan Peerson for biostatistical support. This study was supported by 1R21 HD063275-01A1 from the NICHD and R40MC04294 from the Maternal and Child Health Research Branch, Dept. of Health and Human Services.

Table 1 - *Socio-demographic Characteristics, Breastfeeding Attitudes, and Early Postpartum Breastfeeding Experiences of English- and Spanish-speaking Latinas*

		English Speaking N=52	Spanish Speaking N=62
Socio-demographic characteristics			
Age*	<25	60%	75%
	25-30	14%	19%
	>30	26%	6%
Born outside of the United States***		11%	100%
Mexican heritage*		79%	94%
High School Education or less***		11%	100%
Enrolled in WIC***		58%	94%
Low Income***		58%	94%
Plans to go to work/school within the year***		90%	46%
Breastfeeding Attitudes			
Prenatal breastfeeding intentions°	Weak/moderate	32%	27%
	Strong	23%	23%
	Very strong	45%	50%
Prenatal breastfeeding self-efficacy^	Low	29%	21%
	Moderate	31%	19%
	High	40%	60%
Breastfeeding among family/friends	Mother breastfed*	68%	88%
	Most/all sister or close female relatives breastfed*	44%	63%
	Most/all close friends breastfed	29%	31%
Early postpartum breastfeeding experiences			
In-hospital formula supplementation		54%	58%
Strong perception that environment is supportive of breastfeeding §***		34%	67%

*p<0.05   ***p<0.001

°*Strength of intentions to provide breast milk as sole source of milk for 1st 6 months (Infant Feeding Intentions scale, Nommsen-Rivers, 2009)*

^ *Breastfeeding self-efficacy scale short form, Dennis, 2003*

§ *Most/all family members supportive of breastfeeding, breastfeeding more convenient than bottle feeding, not embarrassed to breastfeed (asked at Day 3 interview)*

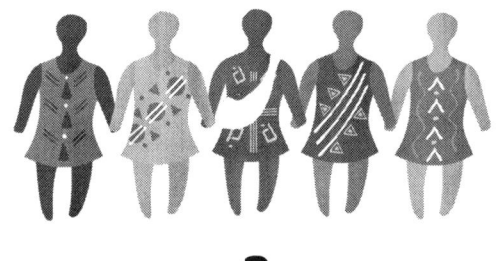

3

Building on Women's Experiences

Brown Mamas Breastfeed—An Analysis of African American Women's Breastfeeding Experiences Shared through an Online Blog Project

Tyra Gross

Breast milk is the most adequate form of nutrition for infants and young children and offers immediate and long-term health benefits for both mothers and children. Health disparities remain persistent in breastfeeding, with Blacks (African Americans) having the lowest breastfeeding rates in comparison to other racial groups (U.S. DHHS, 2010). Very few studies have been conducted examining characteristics of women, especially Black women, who have breastfed despite having risk factors associated with not breastfeeding (Ma & Magnus, 2012). In a breastfeeding study on WIC mothers, Ma and Magnus (2012) concluded that qualitative research is needed to complement quantitative research to examine characteristics of breastfeeding Black women.

While breastfeeding rates have increased for African Americans in recent years, so has the use of social media. Social media is increasingly being used for gathering and communicating health information, such as breastfeeding. Sweet and Simons (2009) state "Health-related blogs ... open up new avenues to communicate information and disseminate research, and they enable 'bottom up' as well as 'top down' exchanges." Although the literature on blogs and health is lacking, a study by West and colleagues (2011) found that blogs are being used to support breastfeeding behavior. Additional research is also needed regarding the utility of blogs for promoting and supporting breastfeeding.

Examining the stories of Black women who have successful breastfeeding experience would fill a gap in the literature and be useful in informing health care providers and public health professionals. This research focused on blog stories specifically written by Black women who have breastfeeding experience. Blogs were selected for analysis because of the availability, cost-effectiveness, and ease of accessing and storing online documents. The purpose of this study is to understand Black women's experiences of breastfeeding documented on blogs. Specifically, what lead participants to the decision to breastfeed their children and

Building on Women's Experiences

how do Black women describe their experiences of breastfeeding?

Methodology

An Internet search was implemented in order to identify suitable blog websites. Google Blog Search engine was used to search blog homepages with the keywords "Black AND breastfeed" in March 2012 (Figure 1). The search was limited to personal blogs with public access, featuring breastfeeding stories from multiple African American women, which were posted since 2010. During the search, an online blog project called *Brown Mamas Breastfeed* (BMB) was discovered. This project was conducted May 2011 on two blogs, *SoulVegMama* and *It's Better at Home*, to highlight experiences of Black mothers who have successfully breastfed their children. BMB will "promote brown mamas sharing and receiving the beautiful gift of breastfeeding" in response to the low breastfeeding rates in the Black community (Jeanine, 2011; Sangodele-Ayoka, 2011).

A call for mothers to submit breastfeeding photos and stories was placed April 2011 on the two blogs with the goal of publishing online for the BMB for Mother's Day 2011. The specific questions asked by the project were: 1) How long have you been breastfeeding? or How long did you breastfeed? 2) Why did you choose to breastfeed? And 3) What do you love about breastfeeding? (Jeanine, 2011; Sangodele-Ayoka, 2011). A total of 23 story submissions were collected from different women. Demographic information was not available for these women, although several mentioned their relationship status and number of children. All stories and photos were collected from the two blogs and entered into a Word document. Although, the photos were retrieved, they were excluded from analysis. Then a table was created to organize the data by name of mother and child, and response to each of the previously mentioned BMB questions.

The constant comparative approach was used to analyze the data. Glauser and Strauss (1967) state that the constant comparative method is a more systematic approach to coding and qualitative analysis, usually to generate theory. The four steps that Glauser and Strauss give for the constant comparative method include the following: 1) comparing incidents applicable to each category, 2) integrating categories and their properties, 3) delimiting the theory, and 4) writing the theory. Although, the goal of this study is not to generate a theory, the constant comparative method will still be utilized to develop codes and derive additional themes from the data.

The first step in analyzing the data was obtaining a sense of the data overall by reviewing all of the data collected. I gathered background information of the BMB from both blogs in addition to all 23 submissions, which included mothers' stories and breastfeeding photographs. The stories were constructed into a table and the photographs were excluded. Secondly, I printed the data table, examined and coded each individual story. With each additional story, I compared and contrasted codes from the previous stories to find patterns within the data. Using pencil, I wrote codes in the margins and drew arrows to connect similarities amongst the stories. I felt that by coding with pencil and paper, I was closer to the data than by coding using the computer. Finally, codes were integrated into larger themes.

Findings

Mothers sharing stories in the BMB had a variety of breastfeeding experiences. The breastfeeding duration for the child currently or most recently breastfed ranged from one month to 27 months. Of the six mothers reporting having multiple children, five had previously breastfed their older children. The longest duration of breastfeeding reported was by a woman who shared: *"all of my babies were breastfed and the longest I have gone is 5 years – twice."* From the 23 stories analyzed from the BMB, several categories developed. In response to first research question, *"How do Black women describe their experiences of breastfeeding,"* the categories were Ongoing Process, Bonding and Nurturance, and Rewards and Challenges.

For the second research question, *"What lead participants to the decision to breastfeed their children,"* the categories were Attitudes, Knowledge and Beliefs, Health and Development, Cost and Convenience, and Social Support. The three overall themes that emerged from the blog stories were 1)

Child Health and Development: *"securing a healthy future for them,"* 2) Fulfilling Experience: "nurtured my patience and potential as a mom," and 3) Importance of Social Support: "no one I knew had done it, and I got little support."

Conclusion

This is the first known study to conduct a blog analysis of Black women's breastfeeding experiences. All women featured in the blogs had initiated breastfeeding. Women shared stories of how long they breastfed, factors that led to their decision to breastfeed, and what they loved about breastfeeding. Racial disparities in breastfeeding practices continue to perplex the public health community. There are gaps in the literature regarding characteristics and experiences of Black women who successfully breastfeed. Despite having the lowest breastfeeding rates in the U.S., African American women are breastfeeding and are choosing so for their children's health and development, and to experience bonding with their children. However, social support from family and health care providers is important and often lacking.

Findings from this qualitative analysis of Black women's breastfeeding experiences shared through blogs can aid public health professionals in implementing effective interventions to decrease the breastfeeding disparity between Black women and those of other races. Decreasing the breastfeeding disparity will subsequently decrease the disparity in infant mortality, and result in improved infant and maternal health for Black women, and the U.S. at large.

Early Infant Feeding Practices among Mothers with High Body Mass Index

Panagiota Kitsantas and Vi Nguyen

The World Health Organization (WHO) has identified childhood obesity as a global public health problem (WHO, 2008). In 2010, U.S. national surveys showed high prevalence rates of obesity in preschoolers (10.4%), school-age children (19.6%), and adolescents (18.1%) (Ogden et al., 2010). There are many factors contributing to overweight and obesity: genetic, metabolic, behavioral, cultural, and socioeconomic. Recent research evidence indicates that maternal pre-pregnancy body mass index (BMI) is associated with offspring obesity and lower rates of breastfeeding (Rooney et al., 2011). Limited information, however, exists about early infant feeding practices among mothers with high BMIs. The purpose of this study was to describe early infant feeding behaviors, including exclusivity of breastfeeding and intensity of breastfeeding at 2-months infant age, and timing of introduction to solid foods in mothers with high BMIs.

Method

Data were obtained from the Infant Feeding Practices Study II (IFPS II), a longitudinal, national survey administered by the U.S. Food and Drug Administration and Centers for Disease Control and Prevention that followed women from pregnancy to one year postpartum. In IFPS II, inclusion criteria required that the infant was born after 35 weeks gestation, weighed at least 5 lbs., was a singleton, and infant did not require hospitalization longer than three days following birth (Fein et al., 2008). The data for prenatal characteristics included 4,814 women. This sample size for this study, however, was reduced to 2,387 for early infant feeding behaviors (2-months infant age) due to follow up loss and missing data on the main variables.

Exclusive breastfeeding, breastfeeding intensity, and adding cereal to baby bottle were assessed based on maternal responses to the 2nd month postpartum survey. Breastfeeding intensity was constructed by averaging the proportion of breast milk to the total milk diet (including breast milk, formula, cow's milk, other milk) that the baby received on a daily basis as reported by the mother in the 2nd month IFPS II surveys. A categorical variable was created with two levels: "low" defined as <20 % of milk feedings being breast milk, and "medium/high" defined as ≥20% of milk feedings being breast milk. Introduction to solid foods was measured based on the mother's report of the age at which her infant was first served solid foods (Li et al., 2008).

Maternal pre-pregnancy BMI was defined as < 19.8-underweight, 19.8 ≤ 26 normal, > 26 ≤ 29-overweight, and > 29-obese. Other variables included mother's age, education, prenatal smoking and gestational diabetes. Whether one of the parents was breastfed as an infant or how the mothers were planning to feed the baby were also assessed based on responses to the prenatal survey. Descriptive statistics, chi-square analysis and logistic regression analyses were conducted.

Results

Table 1 presents the distribution of prenatal characteristics and infant feeding behaviors by maternal pre-pregnancy BMI. We observed that a significantly higher proportion of women with BMIs >29 were at least 34 years old (17.1%) at the time of their pregnancy. High-BMI mothers were less likely to have 4-year college education or more. Gestational diabetes was significantly more prevalent (11.9%) among the women with BMI >29 compared to normal BMI women (4.0%). About 54% of the mothers with BMIs >29 indicated that they were planning to breastfeed their babies, and this was significantly lower than normal BMI mothers (60.4%). A significantly lower proportion of mothers with high BMIs were breastfeeding exclusively at 2-months infant age (36.1%). Further, a significantly higher proportion of mothers with BMIs >29 were breastfeeding at low intensity (38.6%) and started solid foods at less than 4-month infant age (33.9%), compared to normal BMI mothers (26.7%

low intensity and 27.9% for solid foods). Mothers with high BMIs were also significantly more likely to add cereal in baby bottle at 2-months infant age.

Logistic regression models that controlled for maternal age, race/ethnicity, education, smoking, and gestational diabetes revealed that mothers with high BMIs were more likely not to breastfeed exclusively at 2-months infant age and add cereal in baby bottle compared to normal BMI mothers (Table 2). Mothers with BMIs >29 were 1.77 (1.43, 2.20) times more likely to breastfeed at low intensity at 2-months infant age and 1.45 (1.17, 1.78) times more likely to introduce solid foods at <4 months infant age than normal BMI mothers.

Conclusions

The findings of this study indicate that maternal pre-pregnancy BMI influences early infant feeding practices. Women with higher pre-pregnancy BMI had a significantly higher likelihood of never breastfeeding, breastfeeding at low intensity, adding baby cereal in the bottle at 2 months infant age, and introducing solid foods to their infants before 4 months compared to normal BMI women. Both pre-pregnancy BMI and early introduction to solid foods have been linked to childhood overweight and obesity separately in previous studies (Gaffney et al., 2012; Seach et al., 2010). In conclusion, infant feeding practices among women with high BMIs fell short of clinical practice guidelines for infant feeding behaviors. Policy interventions should promote early health infant feeding practices, particularly in mothers with higher BMIs.

Table 1 - *Distribution of Prenatal Sample Characteristics and Early Infant Feeding Practices by Maternal Pre-pregnancy BMI*

Characteristics	BMI < 19.8%	BMI 19.8-25.8%	BMI 26-28.8%	BMI > 29%	P-value
Mother's Age					0.00
18-24 years	39.0	28.4	30.3	21.8	
25-34 years	50.6	57.5	55.1	61.1	
≥ 34 years	10.4	14.1	14.6	17.1	
Mother's education					0.00
High school or less	29.0	22.6	24.4	26.6	
Some college	39.4	39.0	43.6	43.7	
4-year college or more	31.6	38.5	31.9	29.7	
Maternal smoking					0.00
Non-smoker	82.2	88.7	89.5	88.3	
Smoker	17.8	11.3	10.5	11.7	
Gestational diabetes					0.00
No	88.9	87.5	84.5	79.0	
Yes	2.4	4.0	6.2	11.9	
Do not know	8.7	8.5	9.3	9.1	
Was parent breastfed?					0.00
Neither were breastfed/Don't know	48.3	48.8	52.4	56.1	
One parent was breastfed	25.6	23.8	26.4	22.7	
Both were breastfed	26.1	27.4	21.2	21.1	

It Takes a Village

How do you plan to feed the baby?					0.00
breastfeeding only	50.7	60.4	57.6	53.9	
Both breastfeeding and formula	26.3	22.6	27.0	26.2	
Formula only	18.2	13.2	11.9	15.9	
Do not know	4.8	3.8	3.5	4.0	
Exclusive breastfeeding at 2-months infant age					0.00
No	58.4	57.1	63.9	69.5	
Yes	41.6	42.9	36.1	30.5	
Breastfeeding intensity at 2-months infant age					0.00
Low	30.3	26.7	30.7	38.6	
Medium/High	69.7	73.3	69.3	61.4	
Added cereal in a baby bottle at 2-month infant age					0/03
No	85.6	88.6	84.2	84.0	
Yes	14.4	11.4	15.8	16.0	
Introduction to solid foods					0.02
<4 months	26.7	27.9	29.0	33.9	
≥4 months	73.3	72.1	71.0	66.1	

Table 2 - *Effects of Maternal Pre-pregnancy BMI on Early Infant Feeding Practices (ORs and 95% CI)*

Mother's prepregnancy BMI	Did not breastfeed exclusively at 2-months infant age OR (95% CI)*	Low breasfeeding intensity at 2-months infant age OR (95% CI)*	Added cereal in infant formula at 2-months infant age OR (95% CI)*	Introduction to solid foods at <4 months infant age
BMI<19.8	1.02 (0.77, 1.35)	1.14 (0.83, 1.58)	1.14 (0.71, 1.83)	0.83 (0.60, 1.16)
BMI 19.8-25.8	Reference	Reference	Reference	Reference
BMI 26-28.8	1.36 (1.06, 1.75)	1.24 (0.94, 1.64)	1.47 (1.01, 2.16)	1.11 (0.85, 1.45)
BMI >29	1.72 (1.41, 2.11)	1.77 (1.43, 2.00)	1.59 (1.17, 2.15)	1.45 (1.17, 1.78)

*Adjusted for maternal age, race/ethnicity, education, smoking and gestational diabetes

It Takes a Village

Breastfeeding Narratives among WIC Participants in Alamance County, North Carolina

Jennifer L. Proto

Mothers in the Special Supplemental Nutrition Program for Women, Infants, and Children (WIC), a diverse, limited-income group, are especially at risk for low breastfeeding rates and poor health outcomes (Ma & Magnus, 2012). A biocultural perspective, which considers the social, ecological, and biological aspects of health issues and how they interact within and across populations, establishes how formula feeding has become the predominant cultural practice in the United States, particularly for low-income women (Wiley & Allen, 2009; Quandt, 1995). Further, the critical medical perspective, which provides an overall picture of how "social life, social relationships, and social knowledge, as well as culturally constituted systems of meaning" (Singer, 1995, p. 81) impact health behaviors, illustrates how breastfeeding has become a moralized public health practice thought to reduce risk (Dykes, 2005).

The critical medical perspective also demonstrates that WIC-eligible mothers, though many realizing the importance of breastfeeding, face a wide array of risk factors ranging from a lack of support and low socioeconomic status to contradicting misconceptions of the program itself (Dykes, 2005; Evans, Labbok, & Abrahams, 2011; Ma & Magnus, 2012; Morrissey, 2010; Walsh, 2012). Previous research exhibits that successful breastfeeding promotion requires multileveled cooperation by many entities, particularly through the coordination of an International Board Certified Lactation Consultant (IBCLC) overseeing breastfeeding peer counselors. Still, many WIC programs see lower breastfeeding rates than the national average (Chapman, Damio, Young, & Perez-Escamilla, 2004; Fiedling & Gilchick, 2011; Ma & Magnus, 2012). Along with this idea, support for the mother is particularly important not only within WIC but in relationships with family members (Cameron, Javanparast, Labbok, Scheckter, & McIntyre, 2012; Shim, Kim, & Heiniger, 2012) and male partners (Mitchell-Box & Braun, 2012).

In exploring how WIC recipients and providers value the program's services through narrative analysis, this study will consider two medical anthropology theories: the biocultural and critical medical perspectives. A biocultural perspective will help to reveal the social, biological, and ecological components of U.S. breastfeeding practices (Quandt, 1995; Wiley & Allen, 2009). On another level, the critical medical perspective will aid in framing U.S. breastfeeding discourse and women's perceptions of breastfeeding amongst the WIC population (Dykes, 2005; Singer, 1995). Further, previously used interventions will be explored in order to see what methods of breastfeeding promotion are proven to work. In an applied manner, the social and biological natures of breastfeeding, society's way of looking at infant feeding practices, and previously used methods of breastfeeding promotion will be compared to how the WIC program in Alamance County, North Carolina operates and how recipients and providers conceptualize the program's services. This analysis will demonstrate how these factors intersect with WIC programming to ultimately influence breastfeeding success or cessation and reveal areas needing improvement.

Method

Between February and March 2013, 12 semi-structured, open-ended interviews were conducted and recorded both in person and over the phone. These interviews included questions framed by the biocultural and critical medical perspectives found in medical anthropology (Singer, 1995; Wiley & Allen, 2009). In order to explore the social and biological nature of breastfeeding, and the decision making process of breastfeeding mothers, questions focused on WIC, means of support, relationships with the child's father and extended family members, and breastfeeding experiences. Collectively, interviews were transcribed verbatim using a program called F5, and Atlas.Ti was used to code for major themes based upon the interview questions and emergent themes.

Characteristics of the Sample

Findings

Essentially, the WIC providers and recipients in this study mostly agreed on how they value and conceptualize the program. The WIC providers tended to have a more sol-

Building on Women's Experiences

id idea, whereas the recipients realized as time continued following their enrollment in the program. Most recipients enrolled in the WIC program due to economic need, but now value WIC services for its relational breastfeeding and nutritional support.

The narratives of WIC recipients and providers relay fairly congruent frames of reference, agreeing that WIC is a valued resource, which enables breastfeeding successes and nutritional improvements (Morrissey, 2010). WIC recipients and providers concur that the program provides significant support through breastfeeding education, particularly by breastfeeding peer counselors, and nutrition information by nutritionists. The prenatal class was thought to be helpful, and calling was found to be effective and appreciated by recipients, especially before and after delivery.

As a result of programmatic components, all participants acknowledged that breastfeeding is best for the baby's health, yet only two acknowledged that it is beneficial for the mother. This evidence supports Knaak's (2010) findings, which outlines that modern U.S. infant feeding discourse strongly supports the importance of breastfeeding for babies' and though to a lesser extent, mothers' health and wellbeing. Further, both recipients and providers valued WIC's component nutrition education, citing understanding what food to eat and why. Many acknowledged that they did not eat well previously, and it was the combination of the vouchers and the information that made them change their diets. This study, however, does not support that the successes of recipients and providers aligned with the positive opinions of their primary physician and their infant's pediatrician (Tenfelde, Finnegan, & Hill, 2011). Instead, WIC filled this void.

Also, through relaying biological information and offering social support, WIC providers mentioned the aspect of teamwork playing an essential role in their clients' successes. A few recipients picked up on this aspect of WIC's mechanism. The two participants who were WIC providers and recipients seemed to have the most attachment to the program and its organization, benefitting from relationships and support five days a week, on personal levels as Kronborg and Kok (2011) suggest. This study demonstrates that all WIC providers are able to share nutrition information and introduce why breastfeeding is important by suggesting small changes and slowly introducing new ideas. Providers also take these steps together, as recipients see the clerk, lab technician, peer counselor, and nutritionist in one single visit.

Collectively, the narratives of both recipients and providers reveal that interdisciplinary, multileveled support is necessary in order to ensure breastfeeding success. Particularly, this study found that including fathers in the breastfeeding support experience is an important area of need. The mobilization of social support, especially with fathers, can increase feelings of self-efficacy, confidence, knowledge, and acceptance of earlier experiences, aiding in breastfeeding maintenance and sustainment (Kronborg & Kok, 2011;

Building on Women's Experiences

Michelle-Box & Braun, 2012; Stremler & Lovera, 2004). Extended family members were integral in the breastfeeding experiences of Latina/Hispanic participants, whereas it was not as strong of an influence White participants, who emphasized male partners over others. This finding makes sense, as infant feeding practices relate to local cultural practices (Dykes, 2005). For those of Latin American countries, breastfeeding is a cultural practice, and extended family members typically encouraged the Hispanic/Latina participants in this study to breastfeed. In contrast, White participants did not cite breastfeeding, but rather formula-feeding, as a cultural practice, and by breastfeeding, they defied U.S. cultural norms.

An IBCLC and breastfeeding peer counselors, which are included in Alamance County's WIC program, enhance the ability of reaching more women and families, and are able to develop continued relationships, especially with male partners, as well as extended family members (Mitchell-Box & Braun, 2012; Stremler & Lovera, 2004). Therefore, WIC providers could play an integral role in implementing the programming to facilitate the inclusion of male partners and extended family members. However, this gap in the Alamance County WIC program could be a funding issue, since larger WIC programs do have such programs. This situation is not unlike many existent breastfeeding interventions, which lack holistic methods to promote confidence among a broad range of women.

Conclusion

Collectively, similar to how previous research indicates, the participants' narratives support the need for multi-leveled support at micro and macro social levels, though they emphasize the importance of the male partner in their experiences as they negotiate risk and battle cultural and biological barriers, as well as their own emotions (Dykes, 2005; Quandt, 1995, Singer, 1995; Wiley & Allen, 2009). This analysis demonstrates how these factors intersect with WIC programming to ultimately influence breastfeeding success or cessation, particularly in how programming can be augmented or increased to include male partners and extended family members. Ultimately, this research provides greater insight into the existing challenges to optimal breastfeeding practices within this population in Alamance County, North Carolina.

This study did have limitations, which future research should address. A wider spectrum of race/ethnicity of WIC providers and recipients, especially Black/African American mothers, is critical since they are at the highest risk for not breastfeeding (Ma & Magnus, 2011; Walsh, 2012). Also, formula-feeding mothers are likely to have a much different experience with WIC, so their perspective could help to improve the breastfeeding programming. Lastly, the narratives of fathers and other family members are critical, as this study demonstrates the need for members of mothers' social networks to be included in WIC programming, and those present in external support networks should be implemented into future research because of their critical influences on mothers' infant feeding choices (Mitchell-Box & Braun, 2012).

The Challenges of Nighttime Breastfeeding in the U.S.

Cecilia Tomori

Despite recent gains in breastfeeding advocacy and the growing prevalence of breastfeeding, bottle feeding with infant formula remains central to cultural assumptions about infant feeding in the U.S. (Hausman, Smith, & Labbok, 2012; Hausman, 2003, 2011). Breasts are often viewed as sexual objects that should not be exposed in public view, even when feeding babies. Furthermore, breastfeeding is frequently perceived to be difficult, inconvenient, painful, and/or disgusting. At the same time, as a result of public health campaigns, most parents now believe that breastfeeding is "healthy" or "good." Together with the numerous structural barriers that hinder breastfeeding, these conflicted cultural ideologies can lead to the perception of breastfeeding as a morally desirable, but unattainable and problematic practice (Tomori, 2014).

Nighttime infant feeding presents additional cultural problems. In the U.S. it is usually assumed that babies sleep alone, in a bassinet for the first few weeks, and then in a crib in a separate room (Jenni & O'Connor, 2005; McKenna, Ball, & Gettler, 2007). Parents are expected to "teach" babies to go to sleep by themselves and to sleep through the night as soon as possible. Babies who sleep according to these expectations are considered "good babies," and, by extension, their parents are seen as "good parents."

In contrast, parents who bring their babies into bed with them are sometimes considered ignorant or negligent, and are presumed to promote an unhealthy attachment with their children and disrupt their relationship with their spouse (Ball & Volpe, 2013; Gottlieb, 2004; Morelli, Rogoff, Oppenheim, & Goldsmith, 1992; Shweder, Jensen, & Goldstein, 1995). These cultural assumptions, based on values of independence, self-sufficiency, and normative sexuality are buttressed by public health recommendations that suggest that solitary sleep is the only way babies can sleep safely (Ball & Volpe, 2013; Gettler & McKenna, 2010; McKenna et al., 2007).

Evolving Sleep Guidelines

Infant sleep has become a particular area of concern with attempts to reduce the prevalence of Sudden Infant Death Syndrome (SIDS). These guidelines, however, also reflect cultural ideologies about infant sleep and feeding (McKenna & McDade, 2005). In the U.S., guidelines have focused on solitary sleep and positioning babies on their backs, with little regard for breastfeeding. When the American Academy of Pediatrics (AAP) published its 2005 guidelines on SIDS, it emphasized solitary but proximate (same room) sleep ar-

Building on Women's Experiences

rangements, but did not acknowledge the role of breastfeeding in reducing the prevalence of SIDS and recommended the use of pacifiers (American Academy of Pediatrics Task Force on Sudden Infant Death, 2005).

The guidelines were challenged by breastfeeding researchers, and clashed with the views of the AAP's own section on breastfeeding (Eidelman & Gartner, 2006). The 2011 guidelines acknowledge the beneficial role of breastfeeding, but sustain the recommendation against "any bed sharing situation in the home or at the hospital" (American Academy of Pediatrics Task Force on Sudden Infant Death Syndrome, 2011, p. 1351).

Infant Feeding and Infant Sleep in a Comparative Anthropological Perspective

The cultural ideologies surrounding infant feeding and sleep in the U.S. create a particularly difficult environment for new parents intending to breastfeed. Indeed, there are growing indications that breastfeeding parents often violate cultural expectations for sleep by bringing their babies into bed with them in order to manage the demands of nighttime breastfeeding (Kendall-Tackett, Cong, & Hale, 2010). My research investigates the cultural context of the challenges of nighttime breastfeeding and the ways in which parents negotiate them (Tomori, 2014).

Anthropologists have questioned the cultural assumptions that underlie recommendations for infant feeding and sleep based on comparative evolutionary, cross-cultural, and historical evidence. Breastfeeding and proximal sleep arrangements have deep mammalian evolutionary roots and, until recently, were the norm for the human species as well (Ball & Volpe, 2013; McKenna et al., 2007). Biological anthropologists have demonstrated that the proximity of the mother and infant facilitates successful breastfeeding and the coordination of maternal and infant sleep (Ball & Volpe, 2013; McKenna et al., 2007). Breastfeeding and sleeping near children was historically common in the U.S., and remains a globally prevalent practice (Apple, 1987; Ball & Volpe, 2013; Jenni & O'Connor, 2005; Stearns, Rowland, & Giarnella, 1996; Wolf, 2001). Cultural concerns about nighttime proximity and breastfeeding are relatively recent phenomena that are not shared among all groups, even in the U.S. (Kendall-Tackett et al., 2010; McKenna et al., 2007)

Research Study

In order to examine how first-time parents, who intend to breastfeed and have the resources to do so, navigate the challenges of nighttime breastfeeding, I carried out 2 years of ethnographic research with 18 middle-class families from pregnancy through one year postpartum in a small Midwestern city (Tomori, 2014). Participants planned to breastfeed for at least 6 to 12 months. All parents purchased specialized sleep equipment to provide a separate sleep surface for their infants. In addition to participant observation and semi-structured interviews with mothers, partners, and their children, I also observed childbirth education classes, hospital childbirth, and breastfeeding practices; interviewed childbirth professionals; trained as a post-partum doula; and kept informed of media coverage of childbirth, infant feeding, and sleep.

Early Parental Challenges: Negotiating Breastfeeding and Separate Sleep

Despite the educational, financial, and emotional resources available to study participants, many families faced significant challenges to breastfeeding, including inadequate support at the hospital, minimal breastfeeding support from a knowledgeable source after returning home, difficulty mastering the new skill of breastfeeding, and breastfeeding problems. The resulting exhaustion was compounded by parents' struggle to settle their babies to sleep in a separate container. New parents found that their babies awakened every time they placed them in their bassinet or co-sleeper, and needed to be picked up and breastfed. The demands of frequent, often near-continuous feeding, and the difficulties of maintaining separate sleep led parents to revise their sleep arrangements. Consequently, most parents brought their babies into their bed for all or part of the night, at least for the first few weeks.

Parental Concerns about Bedsharing

While bedsharing made breastfeeding and getting rest easier, many parents were concerned about the possibility of harming—and even killing—their babies because of bedsharing. Moreover, many felt guilty about their failure to follow sleep guidelines, their inability to figure out how to get their baby to sleep on her own, and about establishing a "bad" pattern of "dependence" that would be hard to break. Several parents kept their bedsharing a secret from their doctors, relatives, and friends for fear of being judged. Due to these concerns, some parents felt uncomfortable with bedsharing, and struggled to devise strategies to reduce their reliance on bringing their baby to bed with them to facilitate nighttime breastfeeding and sleep.

Negotiating Breastfeeding and Evolving Sleep Arrangements

As babies aged, breastfeeding and sleep arrangements continued to be revised. For several parents, frequent night-waking and breastfeeding disrupted sleep for mothers and spouses, and conflicted with the demands of work schedules. Some parents responded by using sleep-training techniques to reduce nighttime breastfeeding and maintain spatial separation, while others shared their beds more often with their babies. Those parents who habitually shared the bed with their babies were often able to sleep through feedings, but they experienced growing pressure to move their babies to cribs, preferable in a separate room, to "train" the baby to "self-soothe" so that they would fall asleep and stay asleep (without any night feedings) on their own. Nevertheless, a group of parents continued to breastfeed and bedshare with their babies without difficulty and renegotiated their own assumptions about nighttime infant care.

Conclusion

Nighttime breastfeeding and sleep arrangements present significant challenges, even for first-time parents who have the resources to be able to meet their breastfeeding goals. Better advice and support is needed for new parents with a more integrative, evolutionary, and cross-cultural perspective on breastfeeding and sleep.

The Challenge of Late Preterm Birth on Realizing Breastfeeding Intentions

Kristin P. Tully, Diane Holditch-Davis, and Debra Brandon

Introduction

Late preterm newborns (34+0 to 36+6 weeks gestational age) account for 70.4% of all premature births and 8.1% of all births in the United States (Martin, Hamilton, Osterman, Curtin, & Mathews, 2013). Late preterm birth is associated with lower rates of breastfeeding, earlier breastfeeding cessation, and more infant feeding-related morbidities than term birth (Ayton, Hansen, Quinn, & Nelson, 2012; Liu, Qiao, Xu, Zhang, Wang, & Binns, 2013; Radtke, 2011; Zanardo et al., 2011). Meier, Patel, Wright, and Engstrom (2013) recently put forward clinical management strategies to address interrelated infant and maternal late preterm lactation obstacles to improve breastfeeding support for this at-risk population.

The objective of our study was to compare the breastfeeding challenges described by mothers of late preterm infants with those of mothers of term infants to better understand their needs.

Method

This observational study was conducted from 2009-2012.

Participants

Mothers delivered their infants in a regional referral birthing center of a Southeastern academic medical center with approximately 3,300 births per year. Term participants were matched to late preterm participants on maternal race/ethnicity and mode of delivery because demographic characteristics have been found to contribute to the breastfeeding disparity between term and late preterm dyads (Demirci, Sereika, & Bogen, 2013). Mothers were excluded from a larger study (Brandon et al., 2011) if they did not have custody of the infant, if the mother's situation would have affected her ability to participate (e.g., age less than 18, history of HIV, psychosis, or bipolar disorder), or if they were non-English speaking. Mothers providing their milk to their newborns, as indicated by their postpartum hospital records, were oversampled. Infants were singletons and their health was not an inclusion or exclusion criterion.

Participants for this analysis were asked specific questions about infant feeding, which were added in the middle of the larger study. Participants completed interviews and questionnaires face-to-face in the hospital after childbirth and via telephone at one month postpartum. Participant demographics by late preterm and term childbirth status are provided in Table 1. Prenatal infant feeding intentions were collected from a subset of 73 of the 105 participants (38 late preterm and 35 term) during the postpartum hospital interview (see Table 1).

Measures

Maternal and Infant Characteristics

Demographic information was recorded on a form completed by the mother. The infant's medical records were reviewed after enrollment and following hospital discharge to obtain data on obstetric history and medical course. Infant feeding practices were assessed based on maternal report.

Breastfeeding Intentions

During postpartum hospitalization, the Infant Feeding Intentions Scale (IFI; Nommsen-Rivers & Dewey, 2009) was used to assess maternal plans for infant feeding practices. Participants responded to five items, with a range of 0 to 4 for each, for a total of 0-20. Greater scores represent more commitment to breastfeeding over time. In a previous study, Cronbach's alpha for internal consistency was .90

and the IFI Scale was correlated with breastfeeding duration (Nommsen-Rivers & Dewey, 2009). Cronbach's alpha for the IFI Scale in this study was .80.

Participants were also asked their level of "comfort with the idea of formula-feeding." Mothers reported from 1 to 4, ranging from 1 (very uncomfortable) to 4 (very comfortable). Nommsen-Rivers et al. (2010) found that comfort with the idea of formula-feeding predicted infant feeding intentions and mediated the disparity in breastfeeding intentions between different ethnic groups of American mothers.

Semi-Structured Interviews

The hospital interview focused on the mother's birth story and her infant's care. The interview began with a global statement asking the mother to tell her story about how she "came to deliver." Questions were worded in a non-leading manner to solicit participant understandings, probes were used to elicit full accounts. At one month postpartum, the interview explored how things had been going with the mother and her infant since the previous interview. This analysis addressed maternal responses to the interview questions about recalled prenatal infant feeding intentions and factors that influenced feeding practices.

Procedure

Following Institutional Review Board approval, a research team member confirmed potential eligibility and the appropriateness of potential participation with the nursing staff. Mothers were approached on the postnatal unit, the day after childbirth or later. Directly after a mother provided written informed consent to participate in the study, or at a time during postpartum hospitalization more convenient to the mother, the demographics form and questionnaires were administered and semi-structured interview was conducted. Each subject was in the study for one month. Participant responses audio recorded, transcribed, and then checked for accuracy. The audio files were destroyed once the transcriptions were checked for accuracy.

Analyses

Maternal Questionnaires and Interviews

Maternal responses about infant feeding plans and practices were entered into a matrix format in relation to participant study numbers and the interview questions for ease of comparison. Initial codes were then used to create thematic categories across all participants (Miles, Huberman, & Saldana, 2013). Codes derived from research questions, such as "has anything influenced the way you are feeding your baby," as well as refinements of the core issues that emerged, such as "breastfeeding as too much work for the infant," which the authors identified through an iterative process.

Statistical analyses were conducted using SAS 9.2. For descriptive variables, between-group mean differences on continuous variables were tested using t-tests or with the

Wilcoxon two-sample test due to a non-normal distribution. Between-group differences in proportions were tested using X^2 or the Fisher's Exact Test, as appropriate. The Wilcoxon two-sample test was used to test the breastfeeding intentions between the late preterm and term groups.

Results

Fifty-seven of the 73 mothers interviewed (78.1%) reported that they planned to exclusively provide their milk for some period of time (28 late preterm and 29 term women). Six of the 73 mothers (8.2%) interviewed reported that they prenatally intended to feed their infants their milk supplemented with formula (3 late preterm and 3 term). Ten of the 73 participants (13.7%) reported that they planned to exclusively formula feed from birth (7 late preterm and 3 term). The late preterm and term groups did not differ on their "comfort with idea of formula-feeding." The groups were also similar on their strength of breastfeeding plans. Comfort with feeding methods and the Infant Feeding Intention Scale total scores are reported in Table 2.

Only 44% of mothers who reported that they planned to exclusively breastfeed did so in the hospital. Fewer late preterm mothers provided any or exclusive human milk compared to the term mothers. There was a significant difference in hospital feeding practices between the late preterm term groups, $X^2=16.79$, df=2, $p=.0002$, with less exclusive human milk provision and more formula supplementation in the late preterm group (Table 3).

Hospital challenges common to late preterm and term infants, from their mothers' perspectives, were maternal childbirth recovery needs, limited infant alertness, uncertainty about hunger and satiety cues, and concerns about milk supply. The late preterm group had extra obstacles in the form of more infant intensive medical treatment, breastfeeding as a greater maternal challenge than anticipated, feeding at the breast as too much work for the newborns, more milk expression, and concern for infants losing weight when they were already "small."

More mothers said they planned to exclusively breastfeed at home than did so in the hospital. However, not many reported achieving this at one month. Health professionals were an important source of support for breastfeeding mothers, but participants described varying advice. Weight checks could be a helpful tool but also a justification for formula supplementation. Only one mother reported utilizing, or even being aware of, donor human milk.

Discussion

This study followed late preterm and term mother-infant dyads from hospitalization to the first postpartum month. Late preterm mothers reported less exclusive and any breastfeeding than term mothers. Beyond the breastfeeding challenges common within both groups, the late preterm population had additional practical and emotional infant feeding obstacles. For example, mothers identified physical separation due to intensive care treatment, and/or their recovery process from delivery, as impeding their breastfeeding relationship. Meier et al. (2013) cautions that these risks, and other factors that are known to contribute to delayed onset of lactogenesis II, may go unnoticed when late preterm infants appear similar to term infants. Wang, Dorer, Fleming, and Catlin (2004) suggest late preterm infants represent an unrecognized population at risk for suboptimal care because they "masquerade" as term infants (p. 374). Late preterm breastfeeding outcomes may be better enabled through individualized care and resources developed specifically for this group (such as Meier, 2010).

Further, when maternal-infant complications, such as viewing breastfeeding as "too much work" for infants, impede effective lactation and/or feeding at the breast, donor human milk should be available and accessible for families. Demand for human milk donations in the U.S. currently greatly surpasses the supply (Updegrove, 2013). Some mothers who supplemented with formula during their postpartum hospitalization planned to transition to exclusive breastfeeding at home, but not many of them reported being able to achieve this practice. Post-discharge health care professionals should be aware that a barrier to breastfeeding is the heightened concern of infant weight gain trajectories among mothers who perceive their infants as having been born "small."

Although our sample was diverse and reflective of the community from which it was drawn, it is limited by the exclusion of families with multiples and of non-English speaking Hispanic mothers. U.S. breastfeeding outcomes systematically vary by maternal ethnicity (CDC, 2013). Our study grouped participants by late preterm and term childbirth status to focus on the role of infant medical needs and maternal perinatal experiences on early breastfeeding outcomes. A strength of the study was that the maternal intentions for infant feeding were assessed and the birth groups did not differ in their plans.

Conclusion

The discrepancy we found between planned and reported breastfeeding outcomes indicates that both late preterm and term mother-infant dyads can be better supported. Interrelated biological, emotional, and practical obstacles may underlie the disparity in late preterm and term breastfeeding outcomes.

Acknowledgments

This research was supported by 2KR251106 from the North Carolina Translational and Clinical Science Institute awarded to Kristin P. Tully and Duke University School of Nursing support to the other authors. The Eunice Kennedy Shriver National Institute for Child Health and Human Development Training Grant 2T32HD007376 funded Kristin P. Tully.

It Takes a Village

Table 1 - *Participant Demographics by Late Preterm and Term Childbirth Groups*

	Late Preterm $n=54$ Mean (SD) or % (n)	Term $n=51$ Mean (SD) or %(n)
% White non-Hispanic	50.9 (27/53)	49.0 (25/51)
% Black non-Hispanic	34.0 (18/53)	25.3 (18/51)
% Hispanic and other	15.1 (8/53)	15.7 (8/51)
%Married*	65.4 (34/52)	45.1 (23/51)
%Public assistance	43.1 (22/51)	41.2 (21/51)
% First-time mother	25.9 (14/54)	31.4 (16/51)
Maternal age in years	29.3 (6.3)	28.1 (5.7)
Gestational age in weeks***	35.8 (0.8)	39.7 (1.0)
% Infant female	50.0 (27/54)	41.2 (21/51)
Apgar at 1 minute	7.4 (2.1)	7.6 (1.9)
Apgar at 5 minutes	8.7 (0.8)	8.8 (0.8)
% Cesarean birth	51.9 (28/54)	39.2 (20/51)
Head circumference at birth in cm***	32.3 (1.8)	34.1 (1.5)
Length at birth in cm***	47.1 (2.8)	50.6 (2.7)
Birthweight in grams	2585.1 (470.6)	3351.3 (428.8)
% <2500	48.2 (26/54)	0.0 (0/51)
% 2501-3000	33.3 (18/54)	21.6 (11/51)
% > 3000	18.5 (10/54)	78.4 (40/51)
% Had any pregnancy complications	3.7 (2/54)	5.9 (3.51)
% No prenatal care	3.7 (2/54)	5.9 (3/51)
% Diabetes	9.3 (5/54)	0.0 (0/51)
% Hypertension	37.0 (20/54)	26.5 (13/49)

	Late Preterm $n=54$ Mean (SD) or % (n)	**Term n=51** Mean (SD) or %(n)
% Antepartum Hemorrhage	3.8 (2/53)	3.9 (2/51)
% Chorioamnionitis	5.6 (3/54)	15.7 (8/51)
% Rupture of membranes prior to delivery	67.9 (36/53)	82.0 (41/50
% Received prenatal steroids*	15.7 (8/51)	2.0 (1/51)
% Received prenatal antibiotics**	62.3 (33/53)	35.3 (18/51)
% Only in well baby nursery**	61.1 (33/54)	88.2 (45/51)
Length of hospital stay in days***	7.0 (11.3)	3.1 (3.6)
%Provided maternal milk at discharge	48.2 (39/51)	51.9 (42/51)

Note. Between-group mean differences on continuous variables were tested using *t*-tests, with the exception of length of hospital stay that was tested with a nonparametric Wilcoxon two-sample test due to a non-normal distribution. Between-group differences in proportions were tested using X^2 or the Fisher's Exact Test, as appropriate. *p<.05; **p<.01; ***p<.001

Table 2 - *Infant Feeding Comfort and Plans by Late Preterm and Term Childbirth Groups*

	Group	N	Mean (SD)	Median	24,75 percentile
Comfort with the idea of formula-feeding	Late preterm	22	3.1 (1.0)	3.0	3.0, 4.0
	Term	28	2.7 (1.1)	3.0	2.0, 3.5
Infant Feeding Intentions Scale, Total Score	Late Preterm	26	16.8 (4.3)	19.0	15.0, 20.0
	Term	27	16.0 (3.8)	16.0	14.0, 20.0

Note. Differences in total scores were tested by late preterm and term groups using the Wilcoxon two-sample test, due to non-normality of data distributions (skewness or kurtosis values >0.90). For the Infant Feeding Intentions Scale, the difference in total score was analyzed among those who indicated any intent to provide their milk (score of >1).

Table 3 - *Infant Feeding Practices during Hospitalization and at One Month Postpartum by Late Preterm and Term Childbirth Groups*

	Group	N	% of Group
Hospitalization*			
Exclusive human milk	Preterm	9/54	16.7
	Term	27/51	52.9
Combination of human milk and formula	Late Preterm	33/54	61.1
	Term	14/51	27.4
Exclusive formula	Late Preterm	12/54	22.2
	Term	10/51	19.6
One Month postpartum			
Exclusive human milk	Late preterm	9/45	20.0
	Term	15/43	34.9
Combination of human milk and formula	Late Preterm	18/45	40.0
	Term	13/45	30.2
Exclusive formula	Late Preterm	18/45	40.0
	Term	15/43	34.9

Note. Differences were tested by late preterm and term groups using X^2. **$p<.01$; ***$p<.001$

It Takes a Village

Expectant Moms Respond to "Risk" and "Benefit" Language in Breastfeeding Promotion: Evaluating the Impact of Language on Efficacy

Lora Ebert Wallace and Erin N. Taylor

Purpose

Advocates of the use of risk language in breastfeeding promotion have argued that the usual language used to describe the superiority of breastfeeding and human milk presents breastfeeding and formula-feeding as two roughly equivalent choices, each with advantages and disadvantages (Slaw, 1999; Wiessinger, 1996). Because this "benefits" language emphasizes the advantages of breastfeeding, rather than the disadvantages of formula-feeding, it is argued, this "benefits" language serves to normalize formula-feeding as the standard method, and positions breastfeeding as an optimal, but not usual, method. Thus, "risk language" (which describes the disadvantages of formula-feeding rather than the advantages of breastfeeding) is argued to be a necessary shift in order to "de-normalize" formula-feeding.

This shift in language is one that has been taken up by some breastfeeding advocates and promoters, and has also influenced health policy. In 2003 the U.S. Department of Health and Human Services (DHHS) made a deliberate move to present risks of formula rather than benefits of breastfeeding (perhaps most famously in an advertisement campaign that was withdrawn). DHHS has referenced data from focus groups conducted by the Office of Women's Health (OWH), which showed that, while most mothers have knowledge about the benefits of breastfeeding over formula, most also believe that formula-feeding is an acceptable method (Kukla, 2006; Merewood & Heinig, 2004). Leading researchers and advocates have argued that the use of "risk" language: (1) is a potentially more-effective strategy for increasing rates of breastfeeding, and (2) is a way to re-position norms regarding infant feeding (see MacNiel, Labbok, & Abrahams, 2010; Smith, Dunstone, & Elliott–Rudder, 2009).

The "risk" strategy has gained currency in the breastfeeding advocacy community over the past decade (Kukla, 2006; Kelleher, 2006; MacNiel et al.,2010; Smith, Dunstone, & Elliott-Rudder, 2009; Wolf, 2007), even though the efficacy of the method has not been evaluated, making this theoretical and policy change a currently-relevant area of research inquiry (see Heinig, 2009, who discusses the issue anecdotally; and also Nommsen-Rivers et al., 2010). "Risk" language strategies are already in use by some breastfeeding promoters; for one such "real world" text in use, see: *http://www.healthykent.org/infanthealth/breastfeeding/bf_resource_card.pdf*.

In 2011, we published results of a study examining how readers assess breastfeeding promotional texts and the impact of differing language upon feeding intent, using a general sample of young adult men and women. Results showed that respondents less favorably assessed text using risk language compared to "benefits" text and that feeding intentionality did not significantly differ between those who read text phrased in terms of "risks of formula feeding," and those who read text describing "benefits of breastfeeding." Thus, the use of risk language may not be an advantageous health promotion strategy. A much-needed extension of that research using pregnant women is the subject of this new project. Our current work assesses the efficacy of "risk language" in breastfeeding advocacy among expectant mothers, including: 1) how the promotional information framed as "risks of formula" compared to neutral language ("benefits of breastfeeding") is viewed by mothers-to-be, 2) if "risk" vs. "benefit" texts impact feeding intent prior to birth and feeding behaviors following birth, and 3) impacts of affiliation/source of the information.

Method

In a quasi-experimental, longitudinal design study, 309 expectant mothers in an online parenting community read and assessed (qualitatively and quantitatively) "risk" or "benefit" texts promoting breastfeeding. The "benefit" text is taken from a national breastfeeding advocacy group, and the "risk" text contains all of the same content, but with the neutral language changed to reflect *risks of formula* rather than *benefits of breastfeeding* (e.g., ". . . those who are formula-fed are sicker ... ", rather than, " ... those who are breast-fed are healthier . . . "). In the first of two questionnaires, respondents assessed texts qualitatively and quantitatively, and reported personal and family demographic information as well as their feeding intent (prior to birth). Following birth, respondents will be asked to complete another questionnaire in order to collect information on feeding methods after birth.

Finding

Most respondents (214 of 309) chose to write comments regarding the texts they read. We conducted open and axial coding and analysis of the qualitative data. Conceptual dimensions in the qualitative data include:

- "already heard this,"
- agreement/disagreement,
- belief the text is "informative" or good info,
- desire for more information in general or
- regarding sources,
- belief that the information is "biased,"
- whether they believe text is effective promotional strategy,
- concern for induction of guilt among mothers,
- belief that the language is too harsh or extreme,

- elicitation of emotion (anger, worry, fear, and inspiration),

- a restatement of the text they read,

- assertion that "not all moms can breastfeed," and

- presentation of contrary info or experience.

Perhaps the most interesting and important quality of respondents' remarks, in their own words, is the degree to which many reflect a complex consideration of various aspects and contexts of infant feeding. For example, mothers expressing support for and intent to breastfeed often also noted that "not all moms can breastfeed." Some questioned the accuracy of health claims in the texts, citing concerns for distinguishing correlation from causation. Finally, many found the "risk" language off-putting, with some concerned for mothers who may be discouraged or shamed if they cannot comply, and others questioning the efficacy of informational methods of promotion.

Regarding risk vs. benefit language, mothers who read "risk" texts reacted more than for benefits text conditions (were more likely to write something, and more likely to show emotion), and were more likely to react unfavorably to the text in some way. This is consistent with our analysis of the quantitative date, with respondents reading "risk" texts significantly more likely to assess text as less trustworthy, accurate, and helpful compared to mothers reading "benefits" texts.

Implications

Hearing and listening to mothers' own voices is essential to feminist, mother-centered advocacy. The qualitative component of our study provides one place for mother's own voices. Our research suggests that a one-size-fits-all breastfeeding advocacy strategy that assumes a knowledge deficit may not be the most effective strategy, and could be counter-productive.

A second potential problem of the risk strategy is the moral question of whether this strategy ought to be employed—is it morally acceptable? See Taylor and Wallace (2012) for more on this moral discussion from a feminist perspective. A mother-centered advocacy approach that provides information in a supportive manner, and does not attempt to convince women to breastfeed for health reasons alone, may be less likely to be rejected by mothers. We call for further investigation of the efficacy of methods used in breastfeeding advocacy and promotion, and for use of strategies that include concern and respect for mothers.

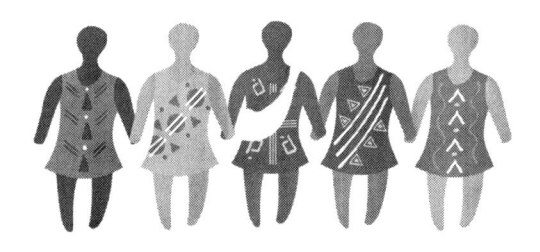

4

Helping Women Integrate Breastfeeding and Employment

Advancing the Breastfeeding-Friendly Campus: Cultivating University Climates can Inspire Change in the Community

Natalie Smith Carlson

Becoming a breastfeeding-friendly workspace is more than the addition of lactation rooms. Nursing mothers need support when the return from maternity leave, set up childcare, and want to share their struggles. We must develop comprehensive programs to address the climate of our businesses and universities, and we should encourage

It Takes a Village

public breastfeeding because of the subsequent agency for mothers, as well as the normalization of natural feeding.

Responding to *The Surgeon General's Call to Support Breastfeeding* requires more than appropriate spaces for natural-feeding mothers to express milk while they are apart from their babies. At North Dakota State University, and places around the nation, we should necessarily advance a climate that promotes best practices for parents and children, and in doing so, set an example that extends into the greater community, inspiring change in attitudes.

We can create this environment by supporting mothers in myriad ways: holding a breastfeeding support group, generating new diversity training, expanding access to childcare, and naming liaisons to prepare for mothers' return to the workplace. As an institution of higher learning, we might even embrace women who breastfeed on campus and how that functions to fracture our androcentric society. Amy M. Saxon (2012), in *The Lactating Body on Display: Collective Rhetoric and Resistant Discourse in Breastfeeding Activism*, highlights the benefits of visual display: "power formations and shifts in the dominant discourse are largely unrecognizable, and yet they work on an individual through subconsciously disciplining both the body and the mind" (p. 17).

The spiraling cycle breastfeeding mothers could institute by nourishing their children, say, in the Union, would lead to expanded notions of normativity and breastfeeding, which could liberate mothers. Saxon uses Barlett (cited in Saxon, 2012) to note, "breastfeeding as a performance rejects the naturalistic argument and allows women agency" (p. 9). The sight of a mother publically breastfeeding on campus would end the invisibility of women who mother and work or study at our university.

Agency is especially significant in patriarchal systems like ours where the call to action is reduced to an issue of space and the (usually men) authority figures assume they just need to grant the rooms and the "problem" will be solved. But, of course, *women* must participate in establishing, evaluating, and promoting a whole program of breastfeeding support! We have been unsuccessfully toiling so long within the existing power structures that are situated around men, "it becomes increasingly obvious that this is not really a question of breast versus bottle, but a question of female embodiment, women's bodies in the public sphere, and the body's potential resistance from within this discourse (pp. 52-53). We understand the imperative of a supportive system on our campus, and we have developed elements that would nurture breastfeeding mothers, and enhance the university climate.

- **Breastfeeding Support Group**

    Our breastfeeding support group sets a precedent for workplaces interested in improving their climates by acknowledging the stress that working and nursing mothers face. Women need a community of strength to value their hard work and we create that at our place of work. *This group could inspire the participants or administrators to create groups beyond campus, and in doing so, will engender an attitude of support for breastfeeding all around the city.*

- **Dedicated Lactation Spaces**

    We have a few dedicated lactation rooms on campus. *More lactation rooms would institute an atmosphere where women expect respectful treatment and then expect the same treatment out in the public world of the city. When students become aware of dedicated lactation spaces, they might realize the possibility of success as a student mother or father—they would feel supported by the university and would enter the workforce expecting more support from the society at large. As happier and more productive parents and providers, they would feel empowered to advocate for breastfeeding.*

- **Lactation Advocates and Allies Program**

    We are working on permission and funding for this program in which partners would identify their support for breastfeeding mothers and display the breastfeeding symbol on their office doors or desks. By including contact information for advocates willing to help parents locate lactation spaces, more people on campus will know exactly who can help them solve any access problems.

- **Annual Employee Training**

  Along with the advocates and allies program, we plan to hold annual training to keep employees of NDSU current about trends and legislation around breastfeeding. *When so many employees are more knowledgeable, they might be more willing to reach out to individuals off campus who need support or solutions.*

- **Diversity Grants**

  As a forward-thinking campus that is building in so many initiatives to propose positive changes, we will be eligible for diversity grants to increase the effectiveness of our attempts. *This could highlight the great climate that we have generated and bring far-reaching attention to the success of our university, and that could inspire other workplaces to work toward the same goals.*

- **Access to Childcare Near Workspaces**

  Women at NDSU have little access to childcare near their work spaces and we must make this improvement a priority. *If it became a standard for women to have quick access to their children, we would see change in the community and women expecting similar working situations. Co-workers would become used to this greater proximity and consider this a right for all nursing mothers.*

- **Breastfeeding Support Information to New Students and Staff**

    Providing information to new students, faculty and staff about our breastfeeding services and programs will help them become enculturated into our supportive system. *This standard may engender an expectation that the support will be the same in the rest of our city.*

- **Liaison on Building Committees**

    A breastfeeding liaison meeting with building committees could help create mother's rooms initially instead of trying to retroactively fit them into new buildings. *Through this, we could see a change in the mentality of construction companies who would advise on other building projects and might expect for lactation rooms to be standard spaces in new buildings.*

- **Liaison Instituting Breastfeeding Plans Before Maternity Leave**

    Working with women to set up breastfeeding support and spaces for nursing and pumping before they go on maternity leave will increase the probability of their success both with breastfeeding and with finishing coursework or remaining happily employed. *Once this is normalized practice, people will begin to expect such considerations for friends and family at all places of work.*

- **Liaison Holding Supervisors Accountable**

    A liaison who seeks out women on campus who need breastfeeding support can facilitate changes with supervisors and spaces around campus. Serving as a protective barrier for mothers who need to make a complaint, the liaison can initiate assessments and work to improve conditions without implicating anyone. *As this person enacts change around campus, he or she might inspire others to take up that role and become liaisons for women in other places in the community.*

We must insist on setting up these new hegemonic power structures in order to design a social situation that cares for breastfeeding mothers. Saxon asks, "What does it mean that she is being asked to cover up or hide in the very establishments where the postfeminist woman has been sold the cultural promise that she may purchase liberation and value?" (p. 22). We must acknowledge the cultural shifts and appreciate the work/life balance that academic, breastfeeding mothers demonstrate for our society. We must construct ourselves into a strong system of support for mothers all over campus by instituting these ideas, keeping women involved, and thanking women for breastfeeding in public.

It Takes a Village

Development of Indicators to Evaluate the Presence of Worksite Breastfeeding Supportive Policies, Benefits, and Environments

Amy E. Meador and Lindsey B. Bickers Bock

North Carolina Prevention Partners (NCPP) has developed a unique web-based strategic planning tool, called WorkHealthy America[SM], to guide workplaces of any size and sector to establish prevention policies, environments, benefits, programs, and practices. This tool is currently comprised of four modules including tobacco, nutrition, physical activity, and creating a culture of wellness. One of the over 120 indicators in this assessment addresses current breastfeeding provisions amongst workplaces.

Breast milk has been identified as the preferred method of feeding for nearly all infants, as it provides health benefits to both the infant and the mother (U.S. Department of Health and Human Services, 2011). The range of health outcomes for both mother and child has been well documented and summarized in the literature. As a result of the positive health outcomes associated with breast milk, *Healthy People 2020* (Office of Disease Prevention and Health Promotion, 2009) has identified "increasing breastfeeding rates" as a national priority with targets of 81.9% of infants being ever breastfed (baseline 74%), 60.6% at 6 months (baseline 43.5%), and 34.1% at 1 year (baseline 22.7%) (Bureau of Labor Statistics, 2009).

Mothers have been identified as the fastest-growing segment of the labor force in the United States (Bureau of Labor Statistics, 2008). In 2008, 56.4% of mothers with infants under 1 year of age participated in the labor force (United States Department of Labor, 2008). This rate is significant, since a woman working outside the home is associated with lower rates of breastfeeding initiation and shorter duration of breastfeeding (U.S. Department of Health and Human Services, 2011). One means of addressing this barrier is to identify ways that worksites can be supportive of breastfeeding, instead of being a hindrance, in order to encourage the initiation and duration of breastfeeding among working mothers.

In 2011, the Centers for Disease Control and Prevention (CDC) contracted with NCPP through the UNC Center for Health Promotion and Disease Prevention (HPDP) to further research the topic and to develop expanded indicators for NCPP's product WorkHealthy AmericaSM related to breastfeeding accommodations.

Method

The existing data collected through WorkHealthy AmericaSM on breastfeeding supportive policies was analyzed to get a snapshot of reported practices. The existing question is worded:

It Takes a Village

Do you provide employees with clean, comfortable, and private areas in which breastfeeding mothers can express their milk during work hours?

This self-reported data on 384 worksites was collected between 2009 and 2013 from worksites that have chosen to participate in WorkHealthy AmericaSM. Users during this period were primarily located in North and South Carolina. As seen in Table 1, this analysis found that 67% of participating worksites provide employees with space and time for lactation. An examination of the demographics of the type of worksites with provisions reveal that larger worksites (77% with over 750 employees, 57% with under 50) are more likely to provide a place for lactation and that non-profit companies (76%) are more likely than either government worksites or for-profit companies (55%).

Creation of New Indicators

The need for breastfeeding interventions in the workplace has been well documented. However, the specific components associated with positive health outcomes are less clear. In order to develop indicators that can help collect evidence to help answer this question, key documents on breastfeeding, and specifically those relating to worksite practices, were reviewed.

Table 1 - *Characteristics of Workplaces Providing Space and Time for Breastfeeding During Work Hours*

	Have provisions *n* (%)	Do not have provisions *n* (%)
All workplaces (N=384)	259 (67.5%)	125 (32.6%)
Hospitals	103 (77.9)	31 (22.1%)
Size (number of Employees)		
0-49	17 (56.7%)	13 (43.3%)
50-99	14 (60.9%)	9 (39.1)
100-249	39 (60.9%)	25 (39.1)
250-749	65 (63.7%)	37 (36.3%)
750+	104 (76.5%)	32 (23.5%)
Structure		
For-profit	64 (55.2%)	33 (44.8%)
Non-profit	119 (76.3)	37 (23.7%)
Government	53 (55.2%)	43 (44.8%)
Education	22 (62.9%)	13 (37.1%)
Note The sample contains a large number of hospitals.		

Examples of references consulted include: *The Business Case for Breastfeeding* by the United States Department of Health and Human Services (2008), *The Surgeon General's Call to Action to Support Breastfeeding* (2011), *The CDC Guide to Breastfeeding Interventions* (Shealy, Li, Benton-Davis, & Grummer-Strawn, 2005), as well as materials by the National Business Group on Health and the United States Breastfeeding Committee. These core documents pointed to many more resources, and others were located using standard search mechanisms in tools, such as PubMed.

It Takes a Village

The information collected from the literature review was used to inform an interview guide designed to solicit expert opinion from experts identified by partners at the CDC. The conversations with the key informants helped pull together concepts from the literature and describe what has been most effective in implementing breastfeeding supportive programs and policies in the workplace. These conversations, based on expert opinion and practical experience, mirrored the information found in the literature, which suggests that in general, breastfeeding support policies are effective for increasing duration of breastfeeding. However, there is sparse research that has been conducted on precisely which elements are most effective in a policy. The experts contacted concurred that the most essential aspects of a formal policy, in their opinion, are provisions for space and time for breastfeeding employees to express their milk or to breastfeed their children.

Based on these findings from the literature and conversations with key informants, indicators to evaluate breastfeeding supportive practices within worksites were created. The questions address the key topics of adequate space and time for a breastfeeding employee to take breaks, written policies, insurance benefits, maternity leave, and options for breastfeeding (as opposed to expressing milk) during the workday. These questions were selected because they promote practices with the highest level of evidence or are promising practices for which more evidence is needed for evaluation.

After the questions were developed, they were field tested with wellness staff at four hospitals. The individuals who field tested the questions also provided us with valuable feedback, which we incorporated into revisions of the questions. Data collection for the revised primary indicator regarding a written policy will begin in summer 2013. The remaining questions will be integrated into a quality of life module still in the development phase, as indicated in Figure below.

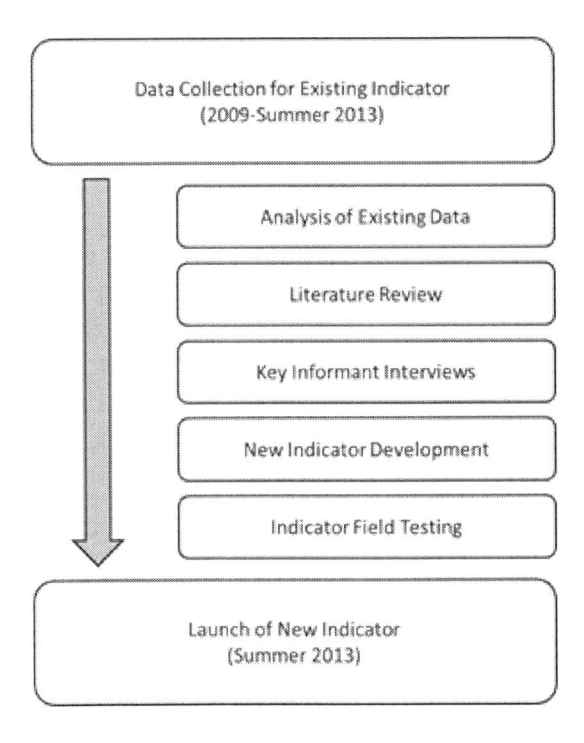

```
Data Collection for Existing Indicator
(2009-Summer 2013)
    │
    ▼
    Analysis of Existing Data
    Literature Review
    Key Informant Interviews
    New Indicator Development
    Indicator Field Testing
    │
    ▼
Launch of New Indicator
(Summer 2013)
```

Figure 1 - *Process for Development of Enhanced Lactation Supportive Indicator in WorkHealthy America[SM]*

Conclusions

The collection of organizational level data through WorkHealthy America[SM] on workplace lactation supportive environments has the potential to help influence the initiation of breastfeeding and/or breastfeeding duration for working mothers by setting a high standard for what is recommended for workplaces to provide their employees. This data, when combined with individual level data sources, also has the potential to contribute to the evidence on what elements of a policy impact initiation and duration of breastfeeding among working women.

Establishing an Employee Lactation Program in a Large Municipal Health Agency.

Yvonne Sinclair, Tamisha Johnson, and Marta Kowalska

In order to achieve individual and public health goals for breastfeeding, accommodations are needed in the workplace for mothers who wish to continue to provide their milk for their babies. In 2008, the U.S. Department of Health and Human Services launched a nationwide initiative called *The Business Case for Breastfeeding*, which presents a toolkit with resource materials and guidelines for establishing workplace lactation support programs. Many models of effective corporate lactation programs are available. However, more examples from diverse worksites can help inform employers of steps in developing and implementing lactation accommodations.

The New York City Department of Health and Mental Hygiene (DOHMH) through its Bureau of Maternal, Infant, and Reproductive Health (BMIRH), oversees a citywide initiative for breastfeeding promotion. The goal of the initiative is to achieve breastfeeding as the normative method of infant feeding. More specifically, the goal is to improve breastfeeding rates in the city, especially for exclusive and longer duration of breastfeeding.

As part of this citywide initiative, the DOHMH launched a lactation program for its own agency employees. The program aimed to help mothers continue breastfeeding upon their return to the workplace, thereby assisting them in meeting their goals for long-term breastfeeding. Additionally, the program sought to set a good example by instituting a service for its own employees that the Health Department's breastfeeding initiative hoped to promote among other New York City employers.

This paper describes the planning and implementation of an employee lactation service for the New York City Department of Health and Mental Hygiene (DOHMH), a municipal agency with a large staff of nearly 8,000. The program offers information about the process, innovative approaches, challenges, and the outcomes of providing a lactation support program in the workplace.

Program Planning Steps

Convene a Planning Group

An Employee Lactation Program planning group was formed from the Wellness at Work committee and was comprised of representatives from several agency units, including human resources, operations, and management. Additionally, several women who had previously expressed a personal interest in provisions for workplace lactation service joined the group. Thus, a diverse and multi-disciplinary group of agency employees was involved in planning the employee lactation program.

Determine the Need for the Program

The planning group requested maternity leave data from the human resources department. The majority of women were from the agency's central office and the others in varying numbers spread across the agency's many work locations. These women had no dedicated lactation facilities or lactation support services at any of the more than 90 DOHMH sites. Since breastfeeding promotion is a priority for the DOHMH, the employee lactation program had approval and support at the highest level of the agency.

Determine What Resources Will be Required

The planning group decided to create a dedicated lactation room in the office building with the most staff requesting maternity leave. However, members were concerned that, because the agency had such a large staff located in several offices citywide, the lactation room alone would not reach a good number of the mothers needing the services. In view of this, the group decided also to have, simultaneously, a loaner pump program, thereby extending the services to employees in other DOHMH locations.

Referrals to community resources would be provided through the BMIRH's Breastfeeding Initiative. To receive employee requests to use the services and to respond to inquiries, an e-mail account was obtained for the lactation service in the agency's email system. Additionally, the BMIRH contracted with a board certified lactation consultant (IBCLC) to provide services on a limited basis. The consultant services included breastfeeding education and clinical counseling for mothers who had breastfeeding questions and concerns, occasional support group sessions, and quality assurance checks on the room and pumps.

Start-up cost of the program was approximately $3,000, which included the purchase of two chairs and a refrigerator for the lactation room, and facilities improvement costs, such as painting of the room and installation of a door lock.

Establish Program Protocols

The employee lactation program was to be implemented as joint effort between the Wellness at Work Program and the Bureau of Maternal, Infant and Reproductive Health, however, the latter agency subsequently assumed full re-

It Takes a Village

sponsibility for the coordination and oversight of the program when the Wellness at Work program ceased operation.

Written protocols were developed for the services. The protocols outlined matters relating to time, access to services, how to participate and other guidelines for the use of the services. The document was then placed on the agency's Intranet in the list of employee resources.

Staff was introduced to the employee lactation program through an agency-wide email announcement. The official launch of the program was commemorated with a ribbon cutting ceremony.

Program Implementation

Facilities and Materials

The NYC DOHMH implemented a lactation program that provided mothers the opportunity to express milk during the workday for later feeding of their infant by offering the following:

1. **Employee lactation room.** This is located in the department's main office. The room provides a private area to express milk. It is a 14'x 9' space and contains two hospital grade multi-user electric pumps, two chairs, and a refrigerator. A portable screen separates the room to make two private areas.

2. **A pump-loaner program**. The initiative sends a rented hospital-grade pump (similar to the ones in the lactation room) to the employee's office on loan. Employees using the loaner service make their own arrangements within their individual worksites for space and privacy to express milk.

3. **Pump-attachment kits**. Provided free of charge by the program to employees using either the lactation room or the pump-loaner program.

Administrative Requirements

Once established, the program required minimal amount of time for administration. Program activities involved ordering supplies, registering participants, sending pump kits to users of the lactation room, and pumps and kits to users of the loaner program. Other activities included record keeping, responding to staff inquiries, oversight of the program and scheduling of support group sessions, and QA visits to the room. Although one person could manage all aspects of the service, different level staff of the breastfeeding initiative has handled different components. The time of each staff was not logged, but it is estimated, that total staff time of approximately seven hours per week would be sufficient to administer the program.

Ongoing Program Costs

Recurring costs are for the rental of hospital-grade pumps and purchase of pump kits. In addition, there has been a minimum cost for lactation consultant fees. The program was able to negotiate rates with the pump manufacturer and obtained a discounted rate, making rental costs minimal. The program elected to rent rather than purchase breast pumps to reduce costs associated with cleaning and maintenance of the equipment. The most costly item is the pump kit, which is purchased for $22 each and given free of charge to mothers. Excluding staff time, the program costs approximately $56 per user.

Program Expansion/Improvement

Though not formally evaluated, we have assessed that the following activities would serve to expand and enhance the program: 1) increased promotion of the benefits of breastfeeding and of the program to staff. This could be accomplished by using established agency activities, including new employee orientation; 2) developing and conducting a formal evaluation to determine the impact of the lactation program in increasing breastfeeding duration, and the net gains for the department in terms of productivity, worker satisfaction and retention, cost containment, and/or other employer and employee benefits; 3) assessment of options for maternity leave, alternate accommodations for nursing mothers, and adoption of policies and practices that are family-friendly and that are supportive of breastfeeding in all work settings, including field work.

Conclusion

The DOHMH has established a workplace lactation program that provides suitable options for nursing mothers. The program has subsequently expanded to include a total of three lactation rooms in two locations, a loaner pump program, a support group, group and individual calls with a lactation consultant, and breastfeeding materials and a website. The Department's experience demonstrates that employee lactation programs can be of low cost and maintenance. Provision of the lactation program also enabled the DOHMH to be in compliance with the NYS Rights of Nursing Mothers to Express Breast Milk in the Workplace law. The program also served to set a good example in a department that has been carrying out broad public health strategies for breastfeeding promotion. Most importantly, the programs help women meet their goals for longer duration of breastfeeding.

5

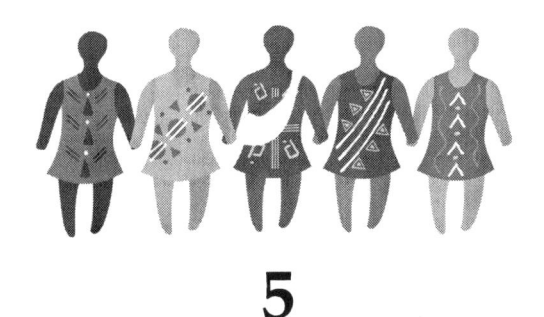

Engaging Communities in Support of Breastfeeding Women

Empowered Communities Ensure Breastfeeding and Good Nutrition of Mothers and Infants

Shobha Arole, Yosef Pandit, Pushpa Sutar, Alison Higgins, and Connie Gates

Since 1970, the Comprehensive Rural Health Project (CRHP), Jamkhed, India, has pioneered principles (equity, integration, and empowerment) and practice of Primary Health Care through comprehensive community-based primary health care (CBPHC). The general well-being and sustained impact on villages has been dramatic, especially of women, children, the poor, and the marginalized, typically the least empowered of the community with the worst challenges for health.

CRHP uses a three-tier system of addressing health in an interrelated, holistic model to address both immediate clinical needs of individuals, as well as assisting the community in taking preventive health and general development measures for the village as a whole. The first tier is at the village level. Highly trained, dedicated volunteer Village Health Workers (VHWs) provide a link to the health team and center, also sharing valuable information and news from the village. They give strong support for initiatives carried out in their village, as well as ensuring that projects originate from the community and are supported by the members of women's and men's groups.

The mobile health team serves as the second tier and the link between the hospital and villages. The team consists of social and paramedical workers, and at times, a nurse and/or doctor. They show support for the VHW within the village, treat cases referred by the VHW, and refer on to hospital when needed, and talk to groups about health and development issues.

The final tier is CRHP's center in Jamkhed, with hospital, training center, and administration. The hospital is equipped to receive emergencies at any time, perform surgeries, serve as an outpatient clinic, and partner with various government and non-governmental organizations

Engaging Communities in Support of Breastfeeding Women

(NGOs) to offer programs, such as eye care and family planning clinics sponsored by others. The training center serves VHWs and community groups as well as thousands of people from government, NGOs, and church organizations, throughout India and the world.

Village Health Workers (VHWs) are a key component of the CBPHC approach. They are the primary change agents, selected by their communities and accountable to them. VHWs are often illiterate and from the poorer classes, making it easy for them to relate to the poorer women, CRHP's target population. They have an enormous amount of training, often years of weekly visits to the center for ongoing training and refresher sessions, after the initial intensive course. The respect they receive from the villagers and knowing that they are making a difference are what motivates them, and very few leave the program once they begin.

VHWs partner with CRHP and are trained in various health topics and personal development. Initially they focus on Maternal and Child Health, a community priority, including breastfeeding, safe delivery practices, prenatal care, counseling, and nutrition. They receive constant support from CRHP in their work and share what they learn with the community, including skills, knowledge, attitudes, and values, through home visits, and with women's groups and farmers' clubs, as well as informally during their daily lives.

It Takes a Village

The VHW helps women and men in the village to organize groups around their own self-interests. Groups serve as the basis for regular learning and sharing about all aspects of health and development, including prenatal care and nutrition, baby care and breastfeeding. Topics covered depend on the goals and interests of the groups and can include water management, treatment and prevention of common illnesses, such as TB and diarrhea, mental health, and agricultural methods. Some women also have organized savings clubs, a form of financial self-help for them. Women also provide peer support and counseling for one another during crisis or to support change.

In CBPHC, through these self-managed groups, villagers are able to build community that works together and is supported in solving problems through identifying challenges and resources, analyzing causes, and developing local solutions. The groups address social situations and other determinants of health, including poverty, caste system, women's and girls' low social status, and those traditional practices that are harmful. The ongoing care and support to the group by the VHW is essential to this sustainable and empowerment process, and her ability to refer problems to the mobile health team and hospital when needed increases the impact even more.

Currently adolescent girls and boys are the focus of special efforts to improve knowledge and attitudes, including nutrition, pregnancy, infant care, to develop capable future mothers and fathers.

Engaging Communities in Support of Breastfeeding Women

Impact on Maternal and Infant Nutrition

Since VHWs know everyone in their village and have good relations, they are aware of pregnancy at an early stage and are particularly attentive to newlyweds. Thus they are able to provide prenatal care including nutrition counseling and support early and throughout pregnancy.

Having a group of women educated and trained in a wide variety of health issues, including the benefits of breastfeeding, helps young mothers separate harmless traditional practices from harmful ones. One particularly challenging tradition related to breastfeeding is the belief that the first milk, colostrum, is harmful to the baby, thereby leading a mother to not breastfeed during the most critical moments of a baby's life, the first three days, giving the baby sugar water instead. Because of the work of VHWs, this practice is today almost non-existent in the CRHP villages, though it holds on in the surrounding communities.

Prenatal care includes checkups at least three times during the pregnancy, and more if there are indications of a problem. Mothers are watched and treated for signs of anemia, hypertension, and other high-risk conditions and referred when necessary. VHWs are also trained to recognize problems, such as a potential breech birth. Pregnant women are counseled about nutrition, especially to overcome traditional food taboos, such as papaya.

The VHW's advice is informed by updated trainings and extends to postpartum care, monitoring the progress of infants and mothers. If there is a feeding problem, for example, a mother not producing enough milk, the VHW ensures the infant gets a natural substitute, such as goat's milk fed with a spoon. Health problems affecting feeding or nutrition, such as diarrhea or pneumonia, are handled at home by mothers or, if necessary, the VHW. Usually, she is with the mother at birth as well, even coming to the hospital with the family if that is what is necessary.

The community supports one another as well, with the men's groups, for example, organizing feeding programs in the early years, including growing nutritious crops, and women's groups developing kitchen gardens. Monthly growth monitoring by VHWs, men's, and women's groups ensures adequate weight gain, identifies problems, encourages and educates mothers about breastfeeding and weaning. As a result, no children from these villages are in hospital due to malnutrition, dehydration, diarrhea, or pneumonia.

Within recent two years (2011 to 2012), in 18 villages, there were 773 live births. Forty (5.2%) were cesarean sections, where the mothers breastfed as soon as possible. Of babies from natural births, only ten (1.3%) were not breastfeeding within one hour. The reasons vary with one maternal death, one premature infant with constant care in a warmer, four twins (two sets) not strong enough to suck, and four mothers with insufficient milk. All others exclusively breastfed for six months and within the first hour.

Conclusion

The CBPHC process empowers a community to act for better health for all, especially women and children, poor, and marginalized. The three-tier system provides an ideal balance between autonomy and support. It is a vibrant and powerful way of assuring support in a variety of health issues, including maternal and infant nutrition. VHWs have the full support of the mobile health team and hospital throughout their work.

The VHW knows her community and can effectively educate about breastfeeding, infant and young child nutrition and common health problems through songs, dramas, role modeling and discussion. She counsels and supports directly and is the person people go to for information regarding health problems, building the respect for the VHW and strengthening her relationship with the villagers over time.

Because of their direct involvement with the mother throughout the pregnancy, their advice on breastfeeding within the hour and exclusively for the first six months carries much more weight. Empowered community members make behavioral changes through understanding and working together. Thus they accept and support breastfeeding, immediate and exclusive for six months, and mothers are also healthy, especially during pregnancy and lactation.

Evaluation of Breastfeeding Peer Support in a Rural Area: What Works for Young, Disadvantaged Women and Their Babies?

Sally Dowling

This evaluation was commissioned by the Public Health Department of NHS Wiltshire, in order to consider how the implementation of breastfeeding peer support (PS) in Wiltshire (a rural county in SW England) might be improved. The focus was three specific areas known to have significant deprivation and low breastfeeding rates. The underlying aim was to consider the effectiveness of PS, how accessible it was to women in these areas, and to those least likely to breastfeed, including young women. Breastfeeding is a public health priority in the UK, widely acknowledged to be important in improving public health. Increasing breastfeeding duration in lower-income groups and amongst younger women is seen as a key target in reducing health inequalities, particularly emphasized by the Department of Health (DH; Dykes, 2005).

Background

Breastfeeding Peer Support

Breastfeeding peer support (PS) is "An approach in which women who have personal, practical experience of breastfeeding offer support to other mothers" (Phipps, 2006, p. 166). Different models include one-to-one (face-to-face and/or telephone) and group support [run by/overseen by the National Health Service (NHS) and/or charities]. The term is usually used to refer to a systematic approach (Kaunonen, Hannula, & Tarkka, 2012), building in a more formalized way on the type of mother-to-mother support successfully offered in the UK by organizations such as La Leche League (LLL), the Association of Breastfeeding Mothers (ABM), and the National Childbirth Trust (NCT). Many peer supporters are volunteers, but there may be a combination of both paid and unpaid, with different degrees of involvement and responsibility.

PS is recognized as an important and effective method of supporting breastfeeding women, as part of a wider strategy within a coordinated program of interventions (NICE, 2008). This necessitates partnership working between a range of statutory, voluntary, and community services. PS is particularly recognized as important in socially deprived communities and in places where breastfeeding is not culturally accepted (Dykes, 2005). The importance of Children's Centres (in the UK) in promoting breastfeeding in these areas has also been recognized (Condon & Ingram, 2011). In addition to increasing breastfeeding rates, benefits of PS may include increased self-esteem and confidence, improving parenting skills, and family diet (Wade, Halning, & Day, 2009), and offering opportunities for increased social contact (Alexander, Anderson, Grant, Sanghera, & Jackson, 2003).

It Takes a Village

Previous evaluations of PS programs (Alexander et al., 2003; Hoddinott, Lee, & Pill, 2006; Ingram, Rosser, & Jackson, 2004) have found them to be effective in increasing breastfeeding prevalence in areas of social and economic deprivation and low breastfeeding rates. Jolly et al., (2012), however, concluded that PS does not increase breastfeeding continuation in higher-income countries, such as the UK. This was suggested to be because of existing postnatal support, and highlighted the need for further research. Antenatal PS and its influence on breastfeeding initiation was examined by Ingram, MacArthur, Khan, Deeks, and Jolly (2010) who conclude that universal PS did not appear to improve rates, although targeted PS may do.

Breastfeeding PS has been funded by the DH in England as part of the Infant Feeding Initiative. An evaluation of 26 DH funded breastfeeding PS projects emphasized the importance of PS in giving positive role models and in enabling the shifting of local cultural norms around breastfeeding (Dykes, 2005).

Breastfeeding in Wiltshire

Work to support breastfeeding in Wiltshire is underpinned by the Wiltshire Breastfeeding Strategy, a three-year plan aiming to increase the number of women initiating breastfeeding, and breastfeeding at 6 to 8 weeks, and to increase breastfeeding at 6 to 8 weeks among women living in the most-deprived communities. This last aim is underpinned by the intention to halve the gap in breastfeeding between women in the least and most-deprived areas in the County. In Wiltshire, DH funding to increase breastfeeding initiation and duration was used to support a number of activities to support the implementation of UNICEF Baby-Friendly Initiative (BFI) Community Accreditation, including establishing and maintaining PS. PS projects were being established in Children's Centers with areas of significantly lower prevalence of breastfeeding, involving ante- and postnatal text and telephone contact.

The Evaluation

The agreed aim of the evaluation was to consider how the implementation of the breastfeeding PS scheme might be improved. The importance of assessing how well recently initiated ante- and postnatal text and telephone contact was working, and whether it was impacting on women accessing PS was also identified. We were asked to focus in particular on PS in three areas in Wiltshire with significant deprivation and low breastfeeding rates, and to consider how accessible it was to women in these areas, and to those least likely to breastfeed, including young women.

The objectives of the evaluation were:

1. To compare how the initiative was working in practice with how it was intended to work.

2. To identify enabling factors for the intervention– both in relation to the context of the intervention and those in the intervention itself.

3. To identify barriers to successful implementation of the intervention.

4. To recommend how to improve implementation of the intervention by developing enabling factors and addressing barriers.

Design and Methods

The evaluation was influenced by realist evaluation (Pawson, 2006, 2013; Pawson & Tilley, 1997) and qualitative methodology. Twelve one-to-one interviews were conducted from May 2012 to February 2013, with a range of stakeholders working in or across the three evaluation areas. These people occupied different positions in relation to the provision of PS. Stakeholders were identified by the commissioner of the evaluation, and health visitor and midwifery managers.

Face-to-face interviews were also carried out with seven breastfeeding mothers. The intention was that these participants were recruited via the PS coordinators in each area. This was straightforward in one area, but problematic in the other. Breastfeeding women were eventually recruited through an alternative route, resulting in interviews with women who had also recently trained as peer supporters. We reflect on the implications of this in our longer report (Dowling & Evans, 2013). Two focus groups were carried out with breastfeeding peer supporters in two out of three identified evaluation areas. Although we were able to speak to two health visitors, no midwives took part in the evaluation.

Findings

Thematic analysis identified five themes: the value of PS, the perception of PS groups, the provision of PS, reaching the women least likely to breastfeed and ante- and postnatal support. These are discussed in depth elsewhere (Dowling & Evans, 2013), supported by extensive quotations from participants. The passion and commitment of the peer supporters was evident throughout. PS was strongly valued for providing social support, as well as help with specific breastfeeding problems. It was seen as normalizing breastfeeding and as providing support, which was often not available, culturally and socially. Women valued the opportunity to meet other mothers who recognized the importance of breastfeeding, and of parenting in this way. Participants recognized that PS was perceived by many as only for those with breastfeeding problems, and for older, "middle-class," or "hippy" women. Groups were not felt to be an appropriate way of offering support to all women, and alternatives were suggested.

PS provided in Children's Centers was sometimes seen as problematic, particularly for those from disadvantaged areas and young women. It appears to work best where there is clear local leadership from someone passionate about breastfeeding, who offers practical and other support to the group and to the peer supporters. PS was not felt to be successfully reaching the women least likely to breastfeed, and this is recognized as a challenging issue. Difficulties include recruiting peer supporters when breastfeeding rates are very low, the need for a range of methods of support, and strongly held family and cultural beliefs about infant feeding. Findings relating to the ante- and postnatal contact intervention were primarily in relation to the importance and value of antenatal contact and the peer supporters' feelings about carrying out this additional role.

Discussion

The findings related to the original objectives of the evaluation. We considered a range of factors that appear to result in few young women and women from disadvantaged communities, accessing PS. These factors included cultural norms and the perception of the groups. During data collection, the planned intervention had not yet been successfully implemented and so we were only able to make some general comments about the perceived importance of this and the implications for peer supporters.

Issues that affect the provision of PS included the location and running of groups, the strong perception of PS groups as being for breastfeeding problems, and the importance for breastfeeding women of the social support they provide. Local leadership was identified as extremely important in the running and maintenance of groups. Examples of good practice in the provision of groups as well as the benefits of PS for the supporters were also highlighted.

Recommendations

A number of recommendations were made to the funders of the evaluation. These include developing a range of models of PS in order to reach women from groups not currently accessing established support; overtly recognizing the importance of groups in providing social support and in providing some elements of lost cultural/societal support; sharing ideas and learning from good practice by contact with those working elsewhere in rural areas and with young women; ensuring that there is appropriate local leadership to enhance the work of the peer supporters and contribute to a supportive infrastructure; engaging in further strategic work in order to fully engage both family doctors and midwives, and recognizing that further work on marketing is needed in order to counter the negative perceptions of groups that prevent some women from accessing support. Further research and evaluation priorities were identified, including an evaluation of the fully implemented text/telephone contact intervention.

This work was carried out in partnership with Professor David Evans, University of the West of England, Bristol, UK. The evaluation was funded by Public Health Wiltshire.

It Takes a Village

From Bottles to Breasts in Rural Haiti

Bette Gebrian and Judy Lewis

Women in Haiti want to be like women in America—their babies fat and smiling, free from illness and, by the late-1980s, bottle-fed. In 1987, few women exclusively breastfed for more than a few days, and less than 1% of them completed 6 months of exclusive breastfeeding (Sabanda-Mulder, 1995). First, a baby was given a traditional purgative (*lok*) on a spoon by grandmothers. Colostrum was expressed and discarded because it "caused diarrhea." The father brought gifts to the home (where most babies were born): meat for the mother and powdered milk or formula for the newborn. "Gerber" was given to babies a few days old if the families had money, and a cracker-based milk and sugar mixture, *labouyi*, if they didn't. The infant mortality was 150/1000.

At the time, the head of the public health program (first author), did not know much about breastfeeding, even though she was educated as a nurse. Training in breastfeeding and the Lactation Amenorrhea Method (LAM) at Georgetown University Institute for Reproductive Health in 1993 shaped the direction of HHF's programs, and made an enormous difference. While all of the training information was practical and useful, critical learning was around three issues: 1) breast milk does not have to be refrigerated; 2) the 3-month growth spurt DOES result in a temporary milk deficit (and a crying baby) that will be equalized with more frequent suckling; and, 3) breast milk is the same quality and quantity, regardless of nutritional status of the mother.

In 1995, UNICEF and the Ministry of Health launched the "Campaign to promote, protect and support breastfeeding" in 20 locations throughout the nation. The Baby-Friendly Hospital Initiative was one component. Education and training was provided to health practitioners and community leaders and families were encouraged to breastfeed for the first 2 years of life. Six hospitals were recognized as "baby-friendly" for not offering baby bottles and encouraging immediate and sustained breastfeeding. But only a fraction of Haitian mothers deliver in hospitals. They deliver at home in both rural and urban areas.

In 1996, the HHF partnered with UNICEF to expand the Campaign's "support" beyond simply talking about breastfeeding to active engagement of pregnant and lactating women, their partners, and their mothers. A type of positive deviance approach was used: women who had breastfed exclusively for 6 months, and fed their babies colostrum, were recruited to be "home visitors." Each mother was "commissioned" to encourage two others in their neighborhood or family to breastfeed exclusively for the first 6 months. They made home visits from the day of delivery through the 6th month. They gave mothers cups with lids and spoons for others to feed manually expressed breast milk when the mother was away. The goal was to reach 1,000 women.

It Takes a Village

Special emphasis was placed on the importance of colostrum and the need to replace *lok*, a purgative traditionally given to newborns. These messages were directed to grandmothers, mothers, and traditional birth attendants. Male partners were given T-shirts when the mother made it to 6 months of EBF (exclusive breastfeeding). Moms and 6-month-old babies, usually fat and happy, were photographed holding the road-to-health card using a Polaroid camera, and the picture was given to them to keep. It was an intense community campaign!

We expected that mothers' work in the fields and markets away from home would be a deterrent to EBF—it was not. One of the biggest barriers was the behavior of nurses, doctors, doctors' wives, and missionary women—they all bottle-fed!

By 1998, an external program evaluation using Lot Quality Assurance Sampling showed that 66% of mothers in villages with health workers, and educated in breastfeeding, breastfed exclusively for 6 months compared to 27% in villages without (Berggren et al., 1998).

The program continued to evolve. Breast pumps were donated for use by nurses and doctors. Breastfeeding bras and clothing were shown (and sometimes given) to women to demonstrate the importance of this behavior. Satisfied mothers became teachers of other women. Wet nursing was initiated for babies of mothers who died in childbirth. Women with breast problems were referred to the clinic for free care. Drivers and other support staff were also trained in breastfeeding support. HHF's computerized health information system was modified to track mothers' use of breastfeeding (complete, partial, or token) each month for the first 12 months.

Lactation consultants from the USA kept us up with current data and best practices. Avera Health System nurses brought belly balls to demonstrate the size of a newborn stomach, more breast pumps, an electric breast pump for the clinic, breast shields, and methods to help pregnant women with inverted nipples prepare for breastfeeding. Their help since 2002 along with the use of HHF villages as public health practicum sites for local nursing students helped to cement this behavior for health professionals and in rural families.

By 2012, women in rural villages served by village health workers and mothers' groups no longer used baby bottles. The purgative *lok* has been replaced by colostrum. Women teach their neighbors, cousins, and sisters how to express milk, keep it cool, and feed it from a plastic cup when the mother is away. They also learn to increase feeding during growth spurts.

Now, thousands of women have exclusively breast-fed their babies for the first 6 months in rural Haiti. They weaned them from 18 to 24 months and increased the space between births to ensure that they and their children have better health.

It Takes a Village

In 2011, HHF was declared the first Baby-Friendly Organization based on UNICEF criteria by the Haitian Ministry of Health. And the first of HHF's 104 villages was designated a Baby-Friendly Village. In 2012, two more villages received this designation.

Reasons for sustainable success?

- Involve the entire village, not just mothers
- Empower mothers to guide each other
- Engage health professionals
- Document the process
- Make home visits often
- Refer problems and assure medical attention
- Reward achievement
- Provide feedback often
- Everyone likes props! Belly balls, bras, photos, an observable sticker on the health cards

Associations between Frequency of Interpersonal Contact Opportunities and Exclusive Breastfeeding Coverage in USAID's Child Survival and Health Grants Program

Kirsten Unfried, Debra Prosnitz, and Jennifer Yourkavitch

While it is clear that mothers need support to optimally breastfeed, the most effective delivery mode and frequency of support remains questionable in different contexts. Various community-based strategies have been developed and evaluated over time. A recent literature review found that more successful approaches are integrated with other interventions that are both acceptable to the community and include active community-based agents (Labbok, 2012)—strategies employed by all of the projects in this analysis.

A meta-analysis of evidence for improving breastfeeding behaviors (Green, 1999) yielded mixed results regarding delivery modes and timing of support. Some suggest that prenatal education in combination with other interventions is associated with improved breastfeeding practices. One study shows that women's support groups lead to positive breastfeeding outcomes. And evaluations of strategies using mass media and print materials are not conclusive. There is more information in grey (project) literature supporting the claim that women's groups have a positive effect on breastfeeding outcomes (Yourkavitch & Lutz, 2010), and a recent paper examining an application of the Care Group model adds further evidence (Davis et al., 2013).

Evidence is mixed regarding postpartum counseling: one study indicates that individual counseling and monthly clinical support together contribute to higher coverage of exclusive breastfeeding (EBF), while another study indicates that counseling and referrals by community-based volunteers do not increase EBF coverage (Green, 1999). A recent meta-analysis concludes that strategies that rely on face-to-face support are more likely to succeed, and support offered reactively—when mothers must initiate contact—are unlikely to succeed (Renfrew, McCormick, Wade, Quinn, & Dowswell, 2012). The authors recommend that mothers be offered support through scheduled visits so that they know when the support will be available and that support should be tailored to contextual needs.

Another meta-analysis concludes that lay support is effective in prolonging EBF (Britton, McCormick, Renfrew, Wade, & King, 2007), indicating that providing effective support is not the province of health professionals alone. The analysis of associations between the type and frequency of community-based interpersonal contacts related to breastfeeding promotion and support and EBF coverage in project areas presented in this paper contributes to the mixed evidence published to date.

For over 25 years, USAID's Child Survival and Health Grants Program (CSHGP) has funded nongovernmental organizations (NGOs) to improve child survival in developing countries. NGOs use a combination of state-of-the-art health interventions and knowledge of local context to design interventions suited to the local populace. Promoting and supporting breastfeeding has been a component of many of these three-to-five year projects, which are implemented in partnership with Ministries of Health and community-based groups.

Projects comprise a variety of strategies, including organizing support groups, educating family members, and training community health workers or lay volunteers to provide direct one-to-one support. These projects also include interventions related to other health areas, including child illness, maternal and newborn care (MNC), and nutrition. In most cases, the same delivery mechanism(s) for breastfeeding support is used for other health behaviors. This analysis examines the association between frequency of interpersonal contact opportunities with mothers through community-based support mechanisms and EBF coverage in CSHGP project areas.

Method

Projects that fit the following inclusion criteria were identified using the CSHGP project database: operated between 2004 and 2011; ended between 2009 and 2011; dedicated effort towards breastfeeding promotion and/or support; and reported baseline and population-based survey data (*N*=30). The authors reviewed project final evaluation reports (available through www.mchipngo.net) and extracted information describing strategies involving interpersonal contacts, which were grouped into six categories: peer support groups (PSGs), regular household visits (HHVs), targeted HHVs (e.g., time-limited visits, such as for antenatal or postnatal care), small group events, outreach services, and growth monitoring/Positive Deviance/Hearth.

Changes in EBF coverage were calculated using baseline and population-based survey data from each project. Statistical significance of coverage changes was determined using a standard formula that assumed 95% confidence. Authors contacted project staff at each organization to verify the extracted data for accuracy and completeness, and to edit or add information, as necessary. Validation was provided by staff from 21 of the 30 projects. Additional project documents were reviewed to fill information gaps. Unless specified, both regular HHVs and PSG meetings were assumed to have taken place monthly, and targeted MNC visits at least once if postnatal care was specified, and at least twice if antenatal and postnatal care both were specified.

Results

Among the 30 projects included in the analysis, 18 reported a statistically significant increase in EBF coverage: 14 of 17 in Sub-Saharan Africa (SSA), three of nine in the

Asia/Pacific region, and one of four in the Latin America/Caribbean region.

Projects used a variety of strategies involving interpersonal contacts to reach their target audiences, of which PSGs and regular HHVs were the most common (20 or more projects each). Notably, all 30 projects implemented PSG and/or HHV strategies, alone or in combination with other strategies.

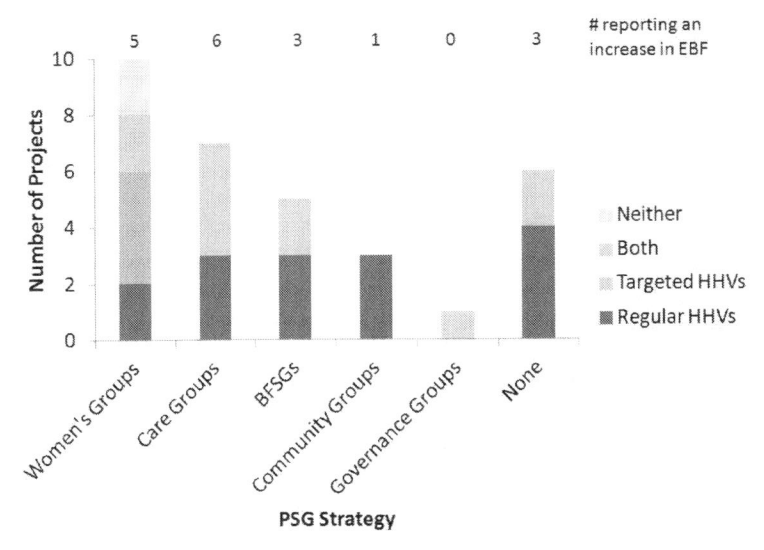

Figure 1

Women's groups were the most common type of PSG used. The Care Group approach (Laughlin, 2004), which, by definition, includes regular HHVs conducted by community volunteers, was the second most common PSG strategy—but was only used in SSA. Other PSG approaches included breastfeeding support groups ($n=5$), community groups (*n*=4), and governance groups (*n*=1). Men's/fathers' groups (*n*=2) and religious groups (*n*=1) were also used—but always in parallel with another PSG strategy. Figure 1 shows the HHV strategies used in combination with PSG strategies, as well as the number reporting an increase in EBF rates by PSG strategy. Projects using Care Groups were the most successful in increasing EBF coverage (6 of 7 projects).

Community health volunteers were the most common type of community-based agent to make HHVs, but in some cases HHVs were made by trained traditional birth attendants or community group representatives.

Discussion

Discerning the frequency of interpersonal contacts for individual women was not possible with available data. Estimating the number of contact opportunities available to a woman over the course of her antenatal, labor and delivery, and lactating periods within the life of a project, occasionally required assuming frequencies of PSG meetings and HHVs, duration of an activity within a project lifecycle, or coverage within a project's target population. These assumptions were reasonably grounded in project descriptions or standard definitions of certain strategies. Attrition and replacement rates of volunteers or group leaders were generally not reported.

Project areas with more than one regular contact opportunity per month through a PSG and/or HHVs were more likely to have increased EBF coverage (Figure 2) and showed a greater average increase in EBF coverage than projects with one or fewer contacts per month ($p=.057$). In this analysis, projects implementing the Care Group strategy showed the best results, consistently, but this strategy has not been widely implemented outside of SSA.

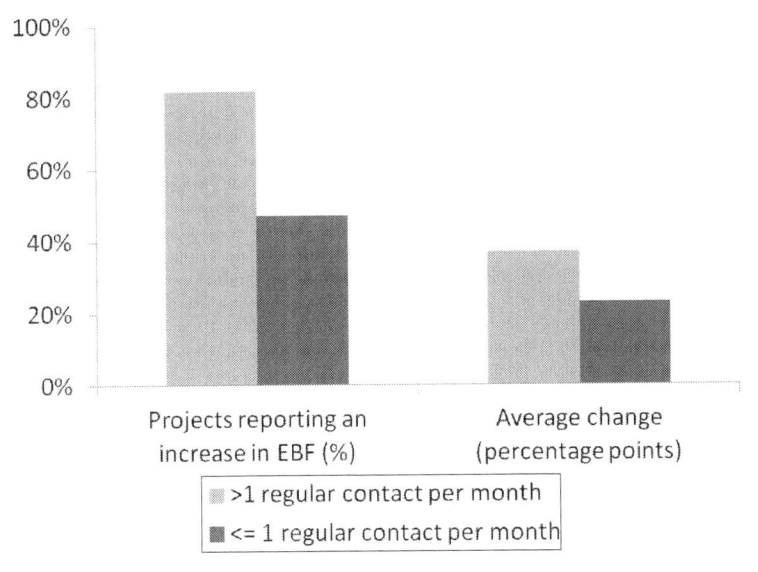

Figure 2

Limitations

This analysis was limited by the small sample size, making it difficult to draw statistically significant conclusions. Project staff were not reachable for all projects, and those that were may have had recall bias. The content of project documents varied. Specific details about interpersonal contact strategies were not consistently reported. The projects were integrated maternal, newborn, and child health projects, and therefore, the level of effort dedicated to breastfeeding among them varied, which may have influenced the changes seen in EBF coverage.

Future Work

To enable estimation of interpersonal contact frequencies across project areas, relevant questions should be developed and incorporated into baseline and population-based surveys. In addition, project staff should describe strategies using a standard reporting template that includes information such as name of strategy, type of community agent, contact frequency, implementation time period, population coverage, and agent training, supervision, support, and attrition/replacement rates. Moreover, detailed cost information would enable "value for money" advocacy and support replication efforts of various interpersonal contact strategies.

Implications

Organizations that want to increase EBF coverage should examine strategies that have worked in similar programming contexts, through published and grey literature, which may be obtained through databases for public programs (e.g., www.mchipngo.net) or by contacting organizations that have promoted breastfeeding in the same (or similar) contexts. In addition, they can access programming guides and tools developed by CORE Group using global evidence and experiences of NGOs. Furthermore, organizations should collect indicators relevant to activities involving interpersonal contacts at baseline and as part of their routine monitoring processes to better understand associations between such contacts and changes in population-level indicators, such as EBF coverage.

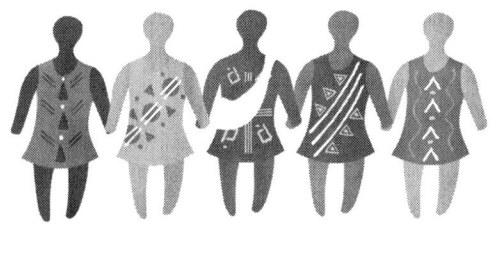

6

Improving Birth Facility and Professional Health Care Support

Lactation Consulting and the Role of Family-Centered Care in Professional Breastfeeding Support

Erica H. Anstey

Part of the challenge in addressing early breastfeeding problems in clinical settings may be that a biomedical approach is child-centered, rather than family-centered, and in this way, the family context and the mother's symptoms (i.e., compressed or damaged nipples) are not often the primary area of concern. In the focused attention on the urgency to deliver enough milk to the child, the breastfeeding relationship can become quickly undermined, especially when the quick fix is supplementation rather than treating or managing the underlying problems(s). Failure to situate the needs of the mother and the family within the context of the solution ignores at least half of the equation. Furthermore, the mother-infant as a dyad may never be assessed by those most likely to be in a position to manage the problem, especially if inter-professional collaboration between providers is tenuous or absent.

Origins of Family-Centered Care

Family-centered care (FCC) is "an approach to health care based on mutually beneficial partnerships among patients, families, and health care professionals" (Johnson, 2000, p. 138). According to the Maternal and Child Health Bureau (MCHB):

> Family-Centered Care assures the health and well-being of children and their families through a respectful family-professional partnership. It honors the strengths, cultures, traditions and expertise that everyone brings to this relationship. Family-Centered Care is the standard of practice which results in high quality services (Maternal and Child Health Bureau, 2005).

The term "family" is variable, and must be understood as such within the context of FCC. The New Mexico Legislature's Task Force on Young Children and Families defines family in this way:

> Families are big, small, extended, nuclear, and multi-generational, with one parent, two parents, and grandparents. We live under one roof or many. A family can be as temporary as a few weeks, as permanent as forever. We become part of a family by birth, adoption, marriage, or from a desire for mutual support . . . A family is a culture unto itself, with different values and unique ways of realizing its dream; together our families become the source of our rich cultural heritage and spiritual diversity . . . Our families create neighborhoods, communities, states, and nations (Johnson, 2000, p. 144).

When considering family in the breastfeeding relationship, the mother-infant dyad is central, but an FCC approach acknowledges that the family is the constant in the child's life, honors the strengths of the family, and respects differences through culturally competent approaches to care.

The concept of FCC dates back to the 1960s, when family advocates began to demand that the traditionally paternalistic health care system make changes to acknowledge the active role of the family as critical to children's developmental and psychosocial needs. This early work led to policy changes that allowed family members to remain with their children during hospital stays and while undergoing procedures. In the 1980s and 1990s, improving the standard of care for children with special health care needs (CSHCN) became a national priority. Various forms of support and legislation, such as a grant from the Maternal and Child Health Bureau (MCHB) in 1985 and the initiation of *A National Agenda for Children with Special Health Care Needs* by Surgeon General C. Everett Koop in 1987, helped to establish FCC as the new standard of care.

In 1992, Family Voices and the Institute for Family-Centered Care (now named the Institute for Patient- and Family-Centered Care) were founded to advance FCC throughout the health care system (American Academy of Pediatrics, 2012; Johnson, 2000; Kuo et al., 2012). As FCC continued to gain popularity in the first decade of the 21st century, many organizations, including the AAP, incorporated FCC into their policy statements. At this time, FCC is widely promoted in many health care settings and has been incorporated into our national health agenda.

Family-Centered Care in Pediatrics

FCC has become the standard practice framework in many health care disciplines, and especially so in pediatrics. The core principles of FCC are (Johnson, 2000):

1. People are treated with dignity and respect

2. Health care providers communicate and share information with patients and families in ways that are affirming and useful

3. Individuals and families build on their strengths by participating in experiences that enhance feelings of control and independence.

4. Collaboration among patients, families, and providers occurs in policy and program development and professional education, as well as in the delivery of care

FCC in the context of pediatrics has been described as:

The belief that health care providers and the family are partners, working together to best meet the needs of the child. Parents and family members provide the child's primary strength and support. Their information and insights can enhance the profession staff's technical knowledge, improve care, and help design better programs and friendlier systems. (Pettoello-Mantovani, Campanozzi, Maiuri, & Giardino, 2009, pp. 16-17).

Much of the literature on FCC in pediatrics focuses on its applicability to children with special health care needs. However, there is some research on FCC in maternity care practices, most commonly related to the NICU experience.

FCC has been widely endorsed as a superior framework for providing effective pediatric health care. However, evidence for the effectiveness of FCC is limited and just beginning to appear in the research literature. The most recent AAP Policy Statement on Patient- and Family-Centered Care (2012) summarizes the positive outcomes of this type of care, as evidenced by the recent literature. These outcomes include fewer emergency room visits, decreased anxiety for children undergoing procedures, faster recovery from procedures, increased satisfaction of care (for the patient and the family), which is directly linked to effective communication, increased confidence and competency for the caregivers, and increased staff satisfaction and cost-effectiveness (American Academy of Pediatrics, 2012).

Despite these promising results, many barriers to the provision of FCC have been identified, including the ability of providers to successfully communicate and negotiate with families to actively incorporate shared decision-making, a lack of coordination, access to services, and patient-provider relationships (Corlett & Twycross, 2006; Gramling, Hickman, & Bennett, 2004; MacKean, Thurston, & Scott, 2005).

Family-Centered Care in Professional Breastfeeding Support

Perhaps due to the relatively nascent field of lactation consulting as a profession, breastfeeding support has yet to be integrated into pediatric FCC practice. FCC is an approach that acknowledges the family as central to the optimal growth and development of the child, and is rooted in the core values of providing collaborative care that respects, engages, supports, and empowers families to build confidence, discover and develop their own strengths, and have a sense of agency in the health care decision-making process.

Pediatrics, maternal and child health nursing, and lactation consulting (IBCLC) all include FCC as a primary philosophy in the standard of care for the profession (American Academy of Pediatrics, 2012; International Board of Lactation Consultant Examiners, 2008; Pillitteri, 2007). Specifically, the scope of practice for the IBCLC includes "using the principles of family-centered care while maintaining a collaborative, supportive relationship with clients" (International Board of Lactation Consultant Examiners, 2008). Though FCC appears to be promoted as the standard of care for each of these professions, it is unclear whether family-centered breastfeeding care is actually being implemented.

Family-centered approaches work within a systems framework, such that the system of care incorporates family-centered principles at the level of the patient, family, community, health care system, and policy. As identified by *The Surgeon General's Call to Action to Support Breastfeeding*, improving breastfeeding success requires a systems approach across the system of care as well (U.S. Department of Health and Human Services, 2011). Inadequate support for addressing early breastfeeding challenges is compounded by a lack of collaboration between providers, such as lactation professionals, nurses, and pediatricians, and the family. Breastfeeding is a biological and sociocultural practice involving many aspects of the health care system, including the breastfeeding dyad, the family, the community, and various health care providers. To implement FCC practices into breastfeeding support, barriers addressing early breastfeeding problems, and barriers to interprofessional collaboration must be identified.

When practicing FCC in professional breastfeeding support, there are several key components of FCC that would apply:

- The mother-infant dyad is at the center.

- The family is respected as the primary caregivers and advocates for their children.

- Culturally competent care respects breastfeeding as more than just a feeding behavior, and honors the many reasons behind a family's decision to breastfeed (or not).

- The family context is considered, which includes various sources of social support, cultural norms, family dynamics including other children, previous experiences, the economic situation, and personal goals, among others.

- The strengths of the family are acknowledged and utilized to empower the family to make decisions.

- The provision of care is flexible to meet the needs of the individual breastfeeding dyad and family.

- Unbiased and accurate, evidence-based information is provided to the mother and other family members.

- Communication and collaboration among providers on the health care team and between providers and community resources is optimally structured to provide the best care possible.

A systems approach is needed throughout the system of health care delivery in the support of breastfeeding to effectively apply FCC. Since little is known about the potential for FCC to be applied specifically to breastfeeding support, more research is warranted. An exploration of the role of lactation consultants as providers of FCC, and their challenges in the context of a health care team, would begin to address some of the gaps in the literature on FCC and professional breastfeeding support.

Application of the Relational Theory to an Academic Program in Maternal Child Health Lactation Consulting: The Transformative Power of Learning

Anna Blair, Karin Cadwell, Kajsa Brimdyr, Cynthia Turner-Maffei, and Beryl Watnick

What is Transformative Learning?

When learning is transformative, the life of the learner is forever changed by not only newfound knowledge, but also by the process of learning. This transformative learning process involves several key components, according to Taylor and Cranton (2012), including that educational offerings must be personally engaging for students and always involve reflection on previous experience. Recognition of the student's embodied knowledge is an empowering element of transformative learning.

Dialogue is also an essential element of transformative learning, although traditional educational approaches (lectures, PowerPoint presentations, etc.) are not excluded from the curriculum as long as the student is engaged and connected to learning and acquiring knowledge. With low residency requirements, our students are able to complete much of the degree online, completing papers after their children have gone to bed or when they get home from work. During their matriculation, students must travel to attend four face-to-face trainings (3 to 5 days in length each), which give them the opportunity to connect with faculty and learn skills (such as assessment and counseling), which are more effectively taught in person. Competencies are verified during the face-to-face courses.

Dialogue includes the fostering of discourse.

Participants need "accurate and complete information; freedom from coercion and distorting self-deception; openness to alternative points of view: empathy and concern about how others think and feel; the ability to weigh evidence and assess arguments objectively; greater awareness of the text of ideas and, more critically, reflectiveness of assumptions, including their own; an equal opportunity to participate in the various roles of the discourse; willingness to seek understanding and agreement and to accept a resulting best judgment as a test of validity until new perspectives, evidence, or arguments are encountered and validated through discourse as yielding a better judgment" (Mezirow, 2012, p. 80).

Creating this environment for open discourse means that students develop critical thinking skills as adults, which may be new, as their previous experiences with secondary education and college may have had a different pedagogical structure.

The information learned in the transformative process is practical in nature: learning that can be applied to real life.

It is not "arbitrary" learning, where "teaching methods are random, ill-defined, and disconnected strategies, with little acknowledgement of their underlying assumptions about learning in general, and more specifically their association with transformative learning" (Taylor & Cranton, 2012, p. 15). Transformative learning acknowledges that learning is not simply acquiring facts but also imagining what else is possible. Solving real-life problems is vastly different than solving mathematical equations: there are often many solutions to explore instead of a single answer. For learning to be transformative, the student's real life must be changed through this exploration. Learning to problem solve involves critical-thinking skills and the consideration of alternative solutions.

If aspiring to facilitate transformative learning, as faculty members we must first acknowledge that although course content is an important part of the learning experience, intuition and personal world view play the crucial role in problem solving. When we are open to the idea that the beliefs that we have held closely could be incorrect, we are then open to possibilities that had previously been unimaginable.

Experts in transformative learning acknowledge that this is a complicated construct. It is especially difficult to describe the connectivity between the student and the information learned because transformative learning does not involve just the memorization of facts that can be assessed by testing, but instead the acquisition of information at a deeper, and more personal level: a life change.

Women's Ways of Knowing (WWOK) and Transformative learning

If learning is to be transformative, the student must be ready to learn—this readiness is key. Many of our students come to the program because they are already in a transformative process engendered by giving birth and breastfeeding, so they are propelled by a desire to be ready. But not every student is actually prepared for the high level of critical thinking and reflective practice expected by the B.S. degree program. For this reason, the undergraduate program was created using the model of Women's Ways of Knowing in order to build the students' readiness for critical thinking, problem solving, and the transformative process.

Transformative learning can be emotional. The path from learning to knowing in real-life situations, with reflective practice, can be challenging. Like the authors of *Women's Ways of Knowing*, we noticed that not all of our learners were coming to the college experience as ideal, ready-to-learn college students, described as having "procedural knowledge, a position in which women are invested in learning and applying objective procedures for obtaining and communicating knowledge" (Belenky, Clinchy, Goldberger, & Tarule, p. 15). Many of our students had been "silenced." Prior experiences with school or birth or breastfeeding (or all three) may have been traumatic or disempowering. The

It Takes a Village

converse could also be true. The new student could be empowered by past experiences to be ready to learn.

By aligning our understanding of the background and developmental trajectory of students in this program, alongside the WWOK model, and the mandatory degree course content, and the university's analytic lenses, were able to fine-tune the learning components of curriculum to allow for the changing needs of students according to the relational model of WWOK, rather than the more classic university expectation that students prove to be "procedural knowers," even before they are accepted to a program.

Curriculum was harmonized so that introductory courses in the major were designed to meet the needs of students who the Relational Theorists would consider women who learn in "silence" or who are "receivers of knowledge." The courses have a lower expectation for problem-solving dialogue and build toward critical thinking as the coursework progresses.

Because many learners come into the MCH program with negative experiences of education and educators, MCH faculty have adopted the conceptual framework described in *Women's Ways of Knowing* as "midwife teachers" who help women give birth to themselves. The faculty try not to be "banker teachers," who expect to deposit information into students' heads. As Stanton reminds us in her chapter in the book of essays, *Knowledge, Difference and Power*, edited by Goldberger, Turule, Clinchy and Belenky:

The task becomes one of discerning the students' individual basis for thinking as they do and finding ways to affirm what they know and how they know it and then finding the means to challenge and stimulate each one to develop more elaborate approaches to the construction of knowledge.

This approach allows students to examine their personal embodied experience as a gateway for engagement in the education process.

Transformation in Practice

Sara Ruddick (1995) argued that maternal work is a discipline. The faculty perspective in the degree programs in Maternal Child Health–Lactation Consulting (B.S.) and Health and Wellness–Lactation Consulting (M.A.) is to agree with Ruddick: helping women to achieve their goals related to lactation and breastfeeding is maternal work, and a discipline. The ultimate goal of both programs is reflective practice, specifically in the area of breastfeeding and human lactation.

The students who were "in silence" may have come to the university only with confidence in their knowledge about how to breastfeed because they did it. Women who are learning in silence may have difficulty in projecting their own "voice," may worry that words are weapons, may want to be obedient to authority, may have grown up in violence and have not been connected to a community. We agree with the authors of *Women's Ways of Knowing* that, in our experience, silenced students "may not have the tools for participating in the kind of discourse community" that have been described by writers and theorists in the transformational learning community. Typically, women who are "silent" learners don't ask questions, are difficult to engage in discussions, and lack confidence in their ability to memorize and retain information.

By acknowledging that some students are not ready for discourse-led problem-solving and critical thinking, we designed the early courses in the program to not only accommodate women learning in silence with straightforward learning experiences, in dialogue mostly with the faculty. In the courses (Anatomy and Physiology, Human Biology, Foundations of Maternal/Child Health, Medical Terminology), students can learn the vocabulary of the field in a non-threatening way so that when they encounter the learning community in discourse and problem-solving later in the program, they will have the requisite confidence in their words and their ability to describe and converse.

The faculty reflected on the framework of *Women's Ways of Knowing* in thinking about students who come to us as receivers of knowledge; women who may be dependent on authority to dispense knowledge. This learner is ready to listen to the teacher's words and wants to show the teacher their new knowledge through return demonstration. We meet these students' needs through the design of our annotated bibliographies and book reviews as assignments that ask for summary, plus critical appraisal in a prescribed format. The summary is often a comfortable task, and the critical appraisal asks them to elucidate the meaning of the work to themselves, and work in the field of maternal child health in general. "Received knowers" learn by taking in knowledge exactly as it is presented and may not be able to integrate competing ideas to acknowledge this learning need, and early courses have been designed so that knowledge is demonstrated through multiple-choice quizzes, which can be retaken without penalty—again, in an effort to allow students to gain confidence that is needed for the transformative process to occur.

Subjective Knowing is another type of knowing described by the relational theorists. When women are learning in this modality, what they know comes from their own experience–in this case, from childbearing, breastfeeding, helping their friends, and being helped themselves. Journaling and online forums give students an opportunity to communicate casually with faculty and other students, and to begin to form community.

The learning needs of students who strongly know subjectively are addressed through open discussion forums. These are important opportunities for students who learn in silence, or as receivers of knowledge, to comfortably participate while learning the vocabulary of the field and gain confidence in their learning readiness. Open-response questions in quizzes and research papers on mid-level course assignments are designed to encourage progression

It Takes a Village

from knowing because I know to knowing through critical thinking and problem solving, and learning as "procedural knowers."

What we see often in the internship phase is a temporary loss of confidence, in the process of transforming to procedural knowing. Students often suddenly realize what they don't know, and what they want to learn, and may become overwhelmed with the enormity of the world of knowledge and evidence within Maternal and Child Health. We also see more active learning and independence in the acquisition of knowledge during the internship. Faculty midwife the students through the internship by individual coaching and supervision, by helping students to understand how to organize ideas using logic and critical thinking, and by offering examples in the use of logic in self-expression.

The student who is a procedural knower is able to acknowledge and give credit to her unique internal voice and use intuition, as well as experts in learning and knowing. The procedural knower is comfortable in dialogue. For the most ready-to-learn student, the constructed knower, the internal voice is unique. Using this voice and negotiating conflicting knowledge, in constructing knowledge, the student can imagine new ways to look at issues. The knowledge she has acquired has become a part of her and she believes that everyone else is capable of constructing knowledge.

In the MCH Program, we expect each student, irrespective of their knowing readiness upon entry to the program, will, by graduation, have transformed into a reflective practitioner.

The student will be able to:

- Learn by doing (how to help mothers/families with breastfeeding, integrating silenced knowing),

- Listen to the experts and perform return demonstrations (integrating received knowledge),

- Learn from experience (integrating subjective knowing),

- Evaluate and apply evidence into practice (negotiating subjective knowing and procedural knowing), and

- Analyze different points of view, question what they have seen or heard, and look for disparities in care with a desire to make positive change.

The transition from procedural knowing to constructed knowing is addressed through clinical placement internships and the capstone, in which students identify a personal interest topic and then address it through the university lenses.

How does the UI&U Maternal Child Health (B.S.) or Health and Wellness (M.A.) program facilitate transformative learning for students who come to the program with a strong voice and confidence in their educational abilities and clinical aptitude? Our program is designed to meet their needs as well. A student who is a procedural knower or constructed knower, upon entry, may find that their experience in the program, as they connect with other students, faculty, and mothers and babies, gives their work new meaning: they believe that every woman can construct knowledge. As they explore the issues of breastfeeding and human lactation through complex lenses they, in turn, develop more clarity about their personal beliefs, ethics, and compass related to evidence-based practice. Our expectation is that our students will all gain greater ability when expressing their beliefs about maternal and child health through the transformative learning process we have designed. We believe that language and voice give power.

If language and voice are where personal power originates, then it follows that connection and conversation are important factors in discovering one's own voice. The challenge, for us, was to create an environment for students to connect with each other in an online arena. Forums built into each unit of the online courses include not only special topics for student discussion for the week/unit, but also provide a place for students who wish to reflect on personal issues. Students who are less ready to connect may only reflect on another's revealing post, without self-revealing at the same depth, and discuss the topic impartially. They may complete the forum posts that are required, and not connect to other students personally at all. For example, we find that some students may ask other students how they

Improving Birth Facility and Professional Health Care Support

arrange childcare during the internship course, while in the same discussion forum, another student reveals the story of her own frustrating breastfeeding experience, of not feeling helped and supported by her partner or family. We cannot fail to be impressed by how students support each other in the forums, even when their opinions differ.

Finding one's voice can be a lifelong work if one is to be a reflective practitioner, which is our ultimate expectation of our students. The first step is to get to know one's self. Rew writes about self-reflection as being imperative in nursing. This is also true for all lactation care providers, whether or not they are nurses.

> Self-reflection is the process of turning one's own thoughts, feelings, beliefs, and behaviors. It is a deliberate process with the goals of discovery and learning. Self-reflection means to look within oneself and listen to the self-talk and associated feelings that guide behavior (Rew, 2009, p. 195).

Our expectation is that self-reflection and evidence are both considered when students examine new research and complex ideas. Motherhood may have started the process of finding one's own voice, and we expect the voice to grow into a powerful and reflective one throughout the academic program.

Hayes and Flannery (2000) explain that women sometimes need to reclaim their voices. They may have had a

It Takes a Village

voice when they were a child or a teenager, but have lost it along the journey to adulthood and parenthood. They may have learned that self-expression is not okay, that it is unacceptable to talk about certain topics or to express certain emotions.

University Analytic Lens for Communication Education: A Means to Finding One's Own Voice

Communication is one of the four university outcomes that are the basis of degrees at Union Institute and University. Written and spoken language skills are built and assessed throughout the program. We know that language is a key element in transformation. Sometimes a course is largely built around the lens of communication. For example, in the course, Folklore in Childbirth, students examine cultural beliefs about birth through story. Writing and reading case studies, and journaling during the internship, writing the capstone, and participating in forum discussions are all means to find voice and communicate.

University Analytic Lens for Critical and Creative Thinking: A Means to Solving Problems

The UI&U programs in lactation require high levels of critical and creative thinking, and are intellectually demanding and require concerted effort and concentration. The expectations of faculty for students are high, but there are barriers. For example, students may come to the B.S. program with considerable transfer credits. With unfinished undergraduate degrees, the concern is about the demands that face women in higher education.

> Women, more so than men, are expected to be constantly available to meet their families' physical and emotional needs. Higher education demands similar devotion of mental and physical energy, along with the ability to separate oneself from the concerns of daily living for concentrated periods of intellectual activity (Hayes & Flannery, 2000, p. 47).

In the online courses, students are able to complete work without needing to be available for "real time" classes. The issue of life demands on students continue, even with the low residency design in place, and some students find that they need to take a term or two off (without penalty) in order to provide more intensive care for their children and/or other family members.

Returning to school after a hiatus is possible. We agree with Hayes and Flannery that it was usually not time-management that was the reason that school was not completed during prior attempts. Women's relationship to her family, friends, and community is the most important aspect of her life: school comes second, third, or last. Even with the unique design of this program, the school/family balance continues to be a challenge for some students.

University Analytic Lens for Social Relevance and Ethics Perspectives: Recognizing Personal Commitment to Service and Social Justice

All of the students in our programs are adults, typically not transitioning directly from secondary school to a university setting, or from a bachelor's degree to the master's degree. Some have partially completed a bachelor's degree. Some have achieved a diploma in nursing. The graduate students have all completed an undergraduate degree, usually not in maternal/child health. Most are driven by a strong personal commitment to ensure that new families receive the breastfeeding care and support they deserve.

Students come to our programs with a deep commitment to support women during birth and breastfeeding. Some come with a positive role model of a Lactation Care Provider who helped during their own breastfeeding experience. Others received little or no support and/or had negative experiences, and come to the program wishing to make sure that others receive the best care possible. Rarely, students who do not have a primary experience with birth or breastfeeding come to the degree programs with secondary experience as a provider of care who wishes to be more knowledgeable and proficient in the care of mothers and babies. As social justice is one of Union Institute and University's university outcomes, issues related to service, social relevance, and disparities of care in this program build on the experiences of students.

Faculty provide assignments that lead to recognition of how social justice and disparities of care are relevant to the Lactation Care Provider, and the capstone provides an opportunity to give further attention and voice to these issues.

University Analytic Lens for Global Perspectives: Finding Our Place in the World

The fourth University outcome provides a focus on the student's place in the world. We expect our students to explore research by diverse populations and about diverse populations. Students examine their own perspective on the world and get a broader sense of their role in their town, their state, their nation, and the international community. By the capstone, students delve deeper to understand the complexity of international health and global maternal/child health issues. This perspective is, of course, valuable if they later decide to work internationally. But a greater understanding of the diversity of beliefs and values can be helpful in all work: local or global.

Reflecting on the Future of the MCH Program

MCH faculty (all women) describe teaching in the UI&U lactation programs as transformational for themselves. Being part of the journey of transformation for the students, also in turn, is transformational. Faculty learn from students, just as students learn from faculty. Faculty make changes every term, based on what is learned from the previous term. The programs have also undergone transformation, as the faculty, advisors, provosts, and deans, as well as outside accreditors have assessed and reassessed throughout the last decade. We know that there is more work ahead and problems which have yet to be solved. Discovering the programs' own voice continues to be a process and a journey.

Summary

"Transformative learning, simply put, is learning that leads to some type of fundamental change in the learners' sense of themselves, their world view, their understanding of their pasts, and their orientation to the future" (Hayes & Flannery, 2000, p. 140). The undergraduate Maternal Child Health: Lactation Consulting degree program and the graduate Health and Wellness Lactation Consulting program at Union Institute and University are transformative for the students and the faculty as we together focus our work on the right of every individual to enjoy good health and have access to care. Having been supported in our own relational development, it is hoped that we are all more prepared to support and foster the transformation in those we all serve: mothers and babies, our students, and each other.

Acknowledgements

The authors would like to thank UI&U Deans, Dr. Carolyn Turner and Dr. Brian Webb, Vice President of Academic Affairs, Dr. Nelson Soto, and Associate Vice President of Academic Affairs, Dr. Elizabeth Pruden, for their continued support of these transformational programs. We also want to express gratitude for the gentle copyediting of Christine Ernst Rathbun.

Low-Income Women's Experiences with Breastfeeding and Lactation Support: A Program Evaluation of a Community Home Visitation Service

Emily A. Dunn

The most vulnerable time for breastfeeding success is the first few days postpartum. The Surgeon General's recent *Call to Action to Support Breastfeeding* (U.S. Department of Health and Human Services, 2011) cites as an example of a breastfeeding barrier the "inadequate assurance of post discharge follow-up for lactation support." Research supports the effectiveness of interventions in the first few days and weeks postpartum. In-home lactation support from a certified lactation consultant, telephone support, and combined professional and peer support all positively affect breastfeeding outcomes (Hannula et al., 2008; Mannan et al., 2008; McKeever et al., 2002).

Low-income women are less likely to breastfeed than middle- or high-income women (Centers for Disease Control and Prevention, 2010; Ryan, Wenjun, & Acosta, 2002). Low-income mothers with the fewest resources have the least ability to overcome breastfeeding barriers (Gross et al., 2011). They experience unique social, political, environmental, and economic circumstances.

It Takes a Village

The Baby Care, a community-based program, provides lactation support services in the early postpartum period to a priority population of low-income, at-risk mothers and infants. These services include phone support, home visits, and electric breast-pump rentals. Ethnographic research methods are utilized to illuminate the lived experiences of low-income women with breastfeeding, and their experiences with lactation assistance postpartum. The study consisted of participant observation and qualitative interviews with recent and current clientele of this home visitation program. All of the participants were receiving WIC, or were WIC eligible. This research seeks to evaluate the program and provide insight into improvement of community-based lactation services for low-income women.

Using biocultural anthropology and feminist theory as a framework, this presentation explores the physical act of breastfeeding within a social context, with a focus on the ways in which biological, political, economic, and social realities are inseparably intertwined. The results consisted of the following main themes: physicality, insufficient milk, nursing in public, pumping, economics, and support.

The main findings of the results presented in this chapter include evidence that this population of mothers may not be receiving adequate support from health care providers, WIC, employers, or family members. This research indicates the cracks that women fall through in health care and social support services. Issues related to economics play a role in the breastfeeding experiences of the women in this low-income population. While mothers may know the benefits of breastfeeding, they did not seem to indicate any worry over dangers of formula-feeding.

Additionally, while mothers express acceptance of others nursing in public, overall they find that doing so themselves is a challenge, and therefore few do so. There is a tradeoff between freedom/autonomy of self and self-sacrifice. Breastfeeding can be a sacrifice of a mother's conception of her body, her time, and her lifestyle. There was little consensus regarding whether lack of success in meeting their lactation goals was due to their personal failure or was the fault of the baby.

One of the main findings was the pervasiveness and impact of the breast pump on the physical, embodied, social, and economic aspects of breastfeeding. Inadvertently, doctors, nurses, and lactation consultants who prescribe the breast pump perpetuate the notion that a mother's body may be inadequate (Torres, 2009). Breast pumps contribute to the medicalization of breastfeeding and emphasize human milk as a product rather than breastfeeding as a process. The breast pump goes along with increasing technological intervention into what was once a normal, non-medical part of life. It perpetuates the mistrust that many women have in their breastfeeding bodies; if the body is a "faulty machine," replace it with a working one (Buckley, 2009).

All of the program participants were grateful for the help that they received, especially since they were often unable to receive pump rental from WIC or elsewhere, indicating that the Baby Café program is meeting mothers' perceived needs. Provision of free lactation consultations and breast pumps remove the financial barrier for women who would not otherwise obtain lactation assistance due to cost. Recommendations for this program are provided based on the evaluation of program processes. These findings can be applied to similar community-based lactation service programs.

These narratives demonstrate the need for community-based lactation assistance programs, but also illuminate structural issues that need to be addressed at larger levels in order to improve the breastfeeding experience for all mothers. A mother without social support and financial resources will be unable to overcome structural constraints that influence the practice of breastfeeding. Breastfeeding cannot be a choice if a mother who chooses to breastfeed is incapable of actually breastfeeding due to policies and practices that impede her choice. Focusing on a woman's right to breastfeed removes the demand from the woman's person and places it on social and political context, "focusing attention on her ability to realize her rights" (Hausman, 2012, p. 19).

A human-rights-advocacy approach to breastfeeding protects the right of the mother/baby dyad to breastfeed by providing an environment that makes breastfeeding possible (though not obligated). In order to create this environment, states must adhere to the International Code of Marketing of Breast Milk Substitutes, promote the Baby-Friendly Hospital Initiative and the Mother-Friendly Childbirth Initiative, implement maternity benefits, and protect breastfeeding in public.

"We Just Have This One Breastfeeding Brochure" (Sponsored by Enfamil): Exploring Breastfeeding Resources and Agenda-Setting in Pediatrics' Offices, WIC, LLL, and the Community Hospital

Katherine A. Foss and Reyna L. Gordon

Outside of La Leche League (LLL) meetings, breastfeeding is an uncommon sight in Middle Tennessee. The absence of public breastfeeding is not surprising, given that Tennessee has the ninth lowest breastfeeding rates in the United States, with only 64% of mothers ever breastfeeding (Centers for Disease Control and Prevention, 2012). Breastfeeding success rests upon an array of complex factors, relating to demographics, individual support, cultural, and institutional determinants (Brodribb, 2010; Humphreys, Thompson, & Miner, 1998; Persad & Mensinger, 2008). Breastfeeding promotional efforts have focused on increasing rates in developing countries or for low-income and/or ethnic minorities in the United States (Ahluwalia et al., 2000; Kaufman, Deenadayalan, & Karpati, 2010; Persad & Mensinger, 2008). Absent from literature on breastfeeding promotion are campaigns that target women across ethnicity, income, and educational levels or studies of available resources in a specific community.

It Takes a Village

This study applied gatekeeping and agenda-setting media theories to study breastfeeding resources in Murfreesboro, Tennessee (McCoombs & Shaw, 1972; Shoemaker & Vos, 2009). Studies on media effects describe how certain authorities serve as gatekeepers of information—deciding what messages are filtered through to the public (Shoemaker & Vos, 2009). Applied to the current research, pediatricians and the proprietors of other health resources control the breastfeeding information locally distributed to the Murfreesboro community. And in agenda-setting, the media (or here—authority figures) do not tell people what to think, but what to think about (McCoombs & Shaw, 1972). In other words, agenda-setting suggests that by focusing on some topics, while dismissing others, doctors and other health professionals convey the degree of importance of particular issues. Using these theories, a textual analysis was conducted on all breastfeeding materials collected or photographed from local health sites. Infant feeding references in "Well Baby Check-up" forms for ages two weeks to 18 months were also examined.

Not surprisingly, the lactation boutique, WIC office, and La Leche League (LLL) offered a wealth of information in English and Spanish. Specifically, the WIC office offered pamphlets on benefits of breastfeeding and how to initiate breastfeeding. They offered to pair this information with feeding videos and a class, and also displayed several posters promoting breastfeeding. The lactation store at the local hospital provided numerous handouts on breastfeeding, all of which were sponsored by a specific pump manufacturer.

On the other hand, the pediatrics clinics lacked such materials, yet promoted other health issues, such as immunization and car seat safety. Only one office distributed breastfeeding information as part of the wellness visit. Two offices offered complementary "for breastfeeding moms" packages, sponsored by a formula brand, which included brief descriptions of breastfeeding benefits, with formula samples and coupons.

Overall, there was a lack of visible and accessible breastfeeding promotional materials, especially at the pediatrics clinics. All the available breastfeeding handouts emphasized the benefits of breastfeeding rather than the risks of formula feeding, and did not necessarily promote breastfeeding as "normal." There was a lack of coordination between local resources: most printed materials did not inform the reader of where to find an IBCLC, how to contact LLL, or where to find other in-person breastfeeding help and support, even though all of these resources exist in this community. Wellness sheets revealed a neutral agenda about breastfeeding in the first few months, and extended breastfeeding was absent from the agenda.

The dearth and poor quality of information at the pediatricians' offices was alarming, given that postpartum support and information dramatically influences breastfeeding success. Such mixed messages can lead to confusion and ambivalence for women, leading to early weaning (Kaufman, Deenadayalan, & Karpati, 2010). The absence of breastfeeding materials and the willingness of the health

It Takes a Village

professionals to display formula coupons may indicate resistance in the local health care community to become more breastfeeding friendly (Bodribb, 2010). For the "Well Baby Check-Up" forms, no reference to breastfeeding appeared after the nine-month form. It was also absent at the 12, 15, and 18 month check-ups.

The scarcity of breastfeeding materials may give insight into the low breastfeeding rates in Tennessee. In the community, the pediatricians and other health professionals serve as gatekeepers of the breastfeeding information—particularly when patients must specifically request brochures and other materials. This gatekeeping function becomes more apparent when the lack of breastfeeding information is paired with the abundance of resources on other health issues. Furthermore, as wellness sheets set the agenda for clinical visits, the neutrality of these forms toward infant feeding early on presents breastfeeding as a comparable health choice to formula, discouraging conversation about breastfeeding obstacles. And the absence of breastfeeding from the forms past age one ignores the notion of extended breastfeeding, possibly causing women to feel ashamed or abnormal if they choose to nurse past this point.

To increase breastfeeding rates, more breastfeeding resources are needed, paired with the removal of counter-messages of formula companies. As modeled by successful campaigns, successful breastfeeding promotion in Murfreesboro must be multi-faceted and overcome resistance from the local health professionals and health care system

(Humphreys, Thompson, & Miner, 1998; Persad & Mensinger, 2008). One important step would be for pediatric offices to adopt the Academy of Breastfeeding Medicine's breastfeeding-friendly protocol (Grawey et al., 2013). Until the cultural climate shifts, breastfeeding in Murfreesboro will primarily exist peripherally, except at LLL meetings.

Growing Breastfeeding Advocates among the Next Generation of Nurses

Jane Grassley

Perinatal nurses are members of the supportive village that inspires and empowers women to initiate and continue breastfeeding. They are in a unique position to introduce new mothers to evidence-based practices that optimize their initial breastfeeding experiences. Unfortunately, nurses' preparation for providing support is often based more on personal experience than current best practices. A lack of education about breastfeeding, particularly in higher education, contributes to nurses' inability to provide evidence-based breastfeeding support, which in turn can adversely affect women's decisions to initiate and continue breastfeeding (Renfrew, Dyson, & Wallace, 2005).

Undergraduate education provides strategic opportunities for introducing future nurses to the importance of breastfeeding and their role in empowering women. The purpose of this paper is to discuss three types of strategies that can be used to facilitate breastfeeding advocacy among the next generation of nurses. These include breastfeeding content within the curriculum, situated learning, and mentoring.

Breastfeeding content can be introduced to all students through a dedicated lecture in a required family, maternity, or obstetrical nursing course. I am invited each semester to present a one-hour lecture to junior nursing students during their family course. I explore with students topics such as what do mother and infants need to breastfeed successfully, nurses' role in creating a positive beginning for breastfeeding, the American Academy of Pediatrics recommendations for breastfeeding, getting the infant latched, assessment of breastfeeding, and breastfeeding challenges.

I teach the students the LATCH tool for breastfeeding assessment, using the online video clips developed by the International Breastfeeding Centre (2012). Although we have not conducted any research to evaluate students' increase in knowledge, students have used this breastfeeding content to develop informational brochures for parents as part of their course requirements.

Other studies have found that providing dedicated breastfeeding content in an undergraduate nursing curriculum can increase students' breastfeeding knowledge (Bozzette & Posner, 2012; Dodgson & Tarrant, 2007). Common content includes the benefits to mothers and children, anatomy and physiology of lactation, position and latch, common breastfeeding complications and management strategies, the nurses' role, the WHO's *Ten Steps to Successful Breastfeeding*, and helpful resources. Basic breastfeeding knowledge is a first step in growing breastfeeding advocates among the next generation of nurses, although knowledge alone does not change students' attitudes about breastfeeding (Dodgson & Tarrant, 2007).

Situated cognitive learning, however, may be more effective in changing attitudes by providing students' with further opportunities to experience breastfeeding advocacy. According to Woolley and Jarvis (2007), situated cognitive learning involves active participation in a clinical environment. I teach a clinical group in a project-based leadership course. During the course of the semester, my senior nursing students collaborate with our community partners at a local hospital to develop projects that support breastfeeding in the NICU and birthing units.

Learning takes place as students review current literature, which introduces them to best practices. They then collaborate with nurse partners using a change framework to develop a real world project that benefits breastfeeding families. The hospital has implemented students' completed projects, which include a learning module for staff about providing skin-to-skin contact between mothers and newborns in the operating room immediately following a cesarean section, and two educational booklets for parents whose infants are in the Neonatal Intensive Care Unit (NICU), one of which gives information about breastfeeding, and one that provides information about breastfeeding after discharge.

The current project focuses on establishing linkages between the local WIC clinic (Women, Infants, and Children Supplemental Feeding Program) and the hospital. These linkages will increase communication and collaboration when infants are discharged from the NICU. Students gain not only more knowledge about breastfeeding, but increased advocacy skills through shadowing one of the NICU lactation consultants and learning about the Baby-Friendly Hospital Initiative.

Their situated learning is further enriched if their concurrent senior preceptor clinical immersion experience takes place in the NICU, in labor and delivery, or on the mother/baby unit. They gain experience with observing how current practices compare and contrast with the best practices they have investigated through the literature. Students feel empowered about their advocacy efforts because the hospital implements their projects.

Other examples of situated learning strategies are case studies (Spatz, 2005) and a comprehensive breastfeeding education intervention that includes 10 hours of didactic breastfeeding content, a skills laboratory, and an 8-week perinatal clinical practicum (Dodgson & Tarrant, 2007). Further advocacy skills are learned in the required advocacy, civic engagement, and policy course in the senior year. Students learn the political process and issue analysis. They write an advocacy paper that they are encouraged to submit to an appropriate legislator. Two students recently wrote papers advocating for a state policy to ban formula gift bags in hospitals. Situated learning, therefore, grows breastfeeding advocates by providing an authentic learning environment where students collaborate with nurses to implement breastfeeding best practices in their clinical settings and learn how to be an advocate (Woolley & Jarvis, 2007).

Mentoring is the third strategy. According to Lisa McKenna (2003), " ... mentoring is a complex, but very powerful relationship between two individuals ... that can provide opportunities for individual to fulfill potential" (p. 7). Each year, I mentor at least one undergraduate research assistant as we investigate breastfeeding support. Through this close one-to-one relationship, students receive socialization into the nursing role of researcher and breastfeeding advocate. My current undergraduate research assistant of two years plans to pursue graduate education as a perinatal mental health practitioner with an emphasis on lactation support. Through participation in a research project exploring adolescent mothers' needs for breastfeeding support, this student gained skills in breastfeeding advocacy as she presented her research at several regional and national conferences.

Undergraduate education provides strategic opportunities for facilitating future nurses' breastfeeding advocacy skills. Students gain knowledge of the importance of breastfeeding for the health of women and children. As they explore best practices for supporting breastfeeding, they are able to critically evaluate and discuss needed changes in hospital environments. Finally, understanding how to facilitate change is a useful advocacy skill as students transition to practice.

The Role of Growth Pattern Interpretations on U.S. Women's Breastfeeding Decisions

Ghada Khan

One of the most frequently cited barriers to breastfeeding continuation among mothers is perceived low milk supply, or perceived milk or breastfeeding insufficiency (Heinig et al., 2006). Recent commentaries have pointed to the association of perceived milk insufficiency with the misinterpretation of breastfed infant growth by health professionals (de Jager, Hartley, Terrazas, & Merrill, 2012). Yet, there has been a lack of formal research regarding this topic. The purpose of this study is to review the evidence surrounding the role of growth chart-based infant growth pattern misinterpretation on perceived milk insufficiency and subsequently, breastfeeding decisions, and to identify gaps in the evidence surrounding this issue.

As the description of this barrier indicates, milk insufficiency is primarily a perceived problem that can stem from the lack of breastfeeding knowledge, understanding, and confidence among mothers (Powers, 1999; United States. Dept. of Health and Human Services, 2011). From a physiological perspective, milk supply is almost always sufficient to support normal infant growth.

Studies that have expanded on the issue of confidence in milk supply have shown that perceptions of milk inadequacy are related to a mothers need to "quantify and visualize breast milk" as a means to gauge their infants health (Dykes & Williams, 1999). One manifestation of breast milk quantification among mothers is enhanced interest in infant growth monitoring and weight gain (Sachs, Dykes, & Carter, 2006). Here, any increase in weight gives a mother the reassurance that breastfeeding is working.

Historically, growth charts have been positioned to represent an empirical, official, and trustworthy referential measure against which infant weight and growth is measured by physicians during routine infant check-ups (Panpanich, Garner, & Logan, 2000), and provide an overall impression for the child being measured [Centers for Disease Control and Prevention (CDC), 2010]. As such, these growth charts are a tangible and official domain against which mothers project their personal perceptions of their milk supply and their breastfeeding successes and failures (Behague, 1993), even though these charts are not meant to serve as a sole diagnostic tool for infant health. Consequently, for some mothers, performance on the chart becomes the most critical indication of their infants wellbeing for which they are willing to give up breastfeeding if this behavior is perceived to threaten optimal performance in any way (Sachs et al., 2006).

It Takes a Village

From 2000 to 2010, providers of pediatric care in the U.S. have predominantly been using growth charts developed by the Centers for Disease Control and Prevention, or CDC growth charts, to assess and monitor infant growth (CDC, 2010). Among the reference population used to develop these charts, 50% of infants were ever breastfed, and only 33% were breastfeeding at three months (Mei, Odgen, Flegal, & Grummer-Strawn, 2008). Prior to that, pediatricians were using the National Center for Health Statistics (NCHS) growth charts, which were based on infants who were predominantly formula-fed (CDC, 2010; de Onis, Garza, & Habicht, 1997). However, studies show that infants predominantly, fully or exclusively breastfed grow differently than those who are formula-fed, and so they do not follow the growth curve represented by the CDC or NCHS growth charts (De Onis, Garza, Onyango, & Rolland-Cachera, 2009; Greer & Bhatia, 2010; Kramer et al., 2004).

Breastfed infants typically tend to be leaner than their formula-fed counterparts during the first year of life, they exhibit differing growth spurts, and are more likely to be misclassified as underweight (De Onis et al., 2009; Mei et al., 2008; Walker, 2011). More specifically, breastfed infants gain weight faster during the first three months than formula-fed infants, but then falter from the CDC and NCHS charts after that (Dewey, 1998; Sachs et al., 2006). Studies show that these differences have led providers of pediatric health care who use growth charts that do not reflect the normal growth patterns of breastfed infants (such as the CDC growth charts), and are unaware of the specific growth patterns exhibited by full-term exclusively breastfed infants to misdiagnose suboptimal growth or underweight among breastfed infants who were actually healthy, feeding well, and gaining weight appropriately.

As small fluctuations from the plotted growth patterns generally decrease, a mother's confidence in breastfeeding is undermined (Sachs et al., 2006). Perceived low milk supply is further perpetuated through this misdiagnosis of suboptimal growth, as this often leads health practitioners to blame breastfeeding inadequacy and suggest unnecessary interventions, such as formula supplementation, or breastfeeding cessation (CDC, 2010; de Jager et al., 2012; Greer & Bhatia, 2010).

In 2006, the World Health Organization launched new Child Growth Standards that established the breastfed child as the norm for assessing growth (World Health Organization, 2008). These standards describe how an infant should grow in optimal conditions, that is, the reference population used to develop these charts were all breastfed for one year, and were handpicked to represent the most favorable socio-demographic and physical environments (CDC, 2010). In recognition of the position of breastfeeding as the best possible standard for infant feeding, in 2010, the CDC, with support from the AAP and the National Institute of Health (NIH) recommended the use of the WHO growth standards in place of the CDC Growth Charts for children under the age of two (American Academy of Pediatrics (AAP), 2012; Centers for Disease Control and Prevention (CDC), 2010).

These recommendations provide pediatricians with the tools to properly assess and monitor the growth of all infants, and not just those who are breastfed. Consequently, the use of the WHO growth standards are predicted to decrease the number of breastfed infants who are categorized as "underweight," and avoid unnecessary interventions that undermine breastfeeding, while also providing a means for the early detection and prevention of overweight among infants who are not breastfed (American Academy of Pediatrics (AAP), 2012). As such, the use of the WHO growth standards has been staged as a means to advocate for the protection, promotion, and support of breastfeeding, and the CDC has developed training modules to help health practitioners understand the differing growth patterns of breastfed infants, and transition to using the WHO charts.

However, there is little evidence surrounding how the use of such charts will affect the growth of exclusively breastfed infants who are reared in suboptimal social and environmental conditions, specifically, environments that significantly differ from those that were used to develop these charts. Here, pediatricians should be encouraged to target and assess the environment where the infant resides in order to make a holistic diagnosis regarding infant feeding.

Evidence is also lacking regarding the implementation of these new charts within the U.S. health system, and there have been few studies dedicated towards understanding how mothers, fathers, and families in U.S. comprehend their application (Panpanich et al., 2000). Consequently, evaluating the uptake of the WHO growth standards, as well as parental knowledge about their use in assessing infant growth, is essential to informing efforts to further breastfeeding support within the area of perceived milk insufficiency among mothers.

The Role of Postnatal Unit Bassinet Types on Enabling Early Breastfeeding

Kristin P. Tully, Helen L. Ball, and Martin P. Ward Platt

The World Health Organization (WHO) recommends that postpartum care include newborns being "in [the mother's] bed or within easy reach" (2006). Mothers and infants remaining together 24 hours a day and encouraging unrestricted breastfeeding are two of the Baby-Friendly Hospital Initiative (BFHI) *Ten Steps to Successful Breastfeeding* (WHO, 2009). BFHI accredited postnatal wards are associated with greater rates of breastfeeding initiation (Bartington et al., 2006; Philipp et al., 2001), exclusivity (Cramton, Zain-Ul-Abideen, & Whalen, 2009; Forrester-Knauss et al., 2013), and duration (Merten, Dratva, & Ackermann-Liebrich, 2005). However, an anthropological lens on mother-infant interactions leads one to question whether standard rooming-in, with a stand-alone bassinet next to the maternal bed, provides sufficient opportunity for extending skin-to-skin contact and enabling breastfeeding (Ball, 2008). Ball states,

It Takes a Village

From both physiological and evolutionary viewpoints, the clinical model of rooming-in as a mechanism for keeping mothers and babies together, and thereby facilitating frequent feeding attempts, would appear less than ideal (p. 133).

Figure 1 - Postnatal Unit Bassinet Types

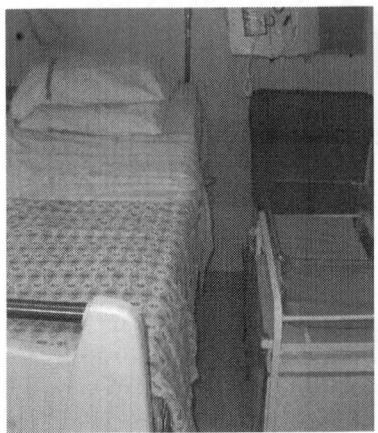

Control, Standard Rooming-in with a Stand-Alone Bassinet *Intervention, Side-car Bassinet Attached to the Bed*

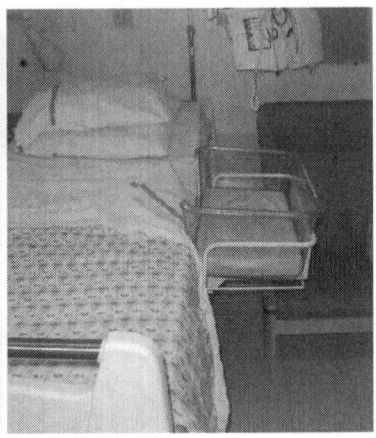

To our knowledge, no research had tested the effects of bassinet types within the rooming-in arrangement on enabling early breastfeeding. Women often have compromised mobility, fatigue, and limited practical support in the postpartum period. Therefore, the stand-alone bassinet that is standard for rooming-in may not comply with the recommendation of having infants accessible, which is critical for early breastfeeding.

Alternatives to the stand-alone (clear acrylic bassinet in a frame on a four-wheeled cart) include bedsharing, or a side-car bassinet that has fits over the side frame of the maternal bed. A flat clamp positioned underneath the mattress locks the side-car in place. The two bassinet types are shown in Figure 1. We conducted two studies to test the effects of the stand-alone bassinet, bedsharing, and the side-car bassinet on postnatal unit breastfeeding frequency and other maternal-infant behaviors.

The prediction was that the frequency of breastfeeding sessions would be greater in conditions of closer proximity (bedsharing or side-car bassinet) compared to the frequency of those allocated to use the stand-alone bassinet. The hypothesis was based on previous research that associated greater breastfeeding with: compact spatial arrangements of home dwellings compared to those that were more dispersed over larger spaces and more floors (Quandt, 1981), mother-infant bedsharing in a laboratory environment compared to the infant sleeping in a stand-alone bassinet in a separate room (McKenna, Mosko, & Richard, 1997), hospital rooming-in with the infant in a stand-alone bassinet next to the maternal bed compared to the infant being in nursery care in a separate room (Yamauchi & Yamanouchi, 1990).

Method

Our team conducted two randomized trials with a parallel design to test effects of bassinet types on facilitating early breastfeeding after vaginal birth (Ball et al., 2006) and cesarean section (Tully & Ball, 2012). In both studies, women were prenatally recruited at a tertiary-level hospital in northeastern England that hosts approximately 5,400 births annually. The maternity unit was not Baby-Friendly Hospital Initiative accredited. Continuous rooming-in with a stand-alone bassinet was standard on the postpartum unit for all healthy dyads.

Ethical and institutional approval were obtained from Durham University and the Newcastle and North Tyneside Research Ethics Committee. In the vaginal birth study, sixty-one women were prenatally recruited, randomized, and filmed with the stand-alone ($n=22$), bedsharing ($n=18$), or side-car ($n=23$). In the cesarean birth study, bedsharing was not an allocated condition due to maternal analgesia and limited mobility. Thirty-five women scheduled for non-labor cesarean were recruited, prenatally randomized, and filmed with the stand-alone ($n=15$) or side-car ($n=20$) bassinet. Recruitment and participant demographics are detailed in Ball et al. (2006) and Tully and Ball (2012).

Both projects entailed filming of mother-infant interactions over the second postpartum night in the hospital. Continuously coded video observations were used to assess breastfeeding, maternal and infant sleep states, midwifery presence in participants' rooms, and infant risk between the trial arms. A taxonomy was used with The Observer (version 5.0, Noldus Information Technology, Wageningen,

Netherlands, May 2003) to categorize behavioral states of mothers and infants, and the presence of midwives.

Observational data were analyzed by a modified intention-to-treat analysis, including all completers. The cesarean study included semi-structured interviews to document maternal experiences with infant care and bassinet use. Participant responses were recorded verbatim, read in their entirety, and entered into a matrix format in response to the interview questions for ease of comparison. Initial codes were then used to create thematic categories across all participants (Wilkinson, 2004).

Results

Ball and colleagues (2006) found that among mother-newborn dyads who underwent vaginal delivery, those who were randomly allocated to have the side-car breastfed more frequently than those allocated the stand-alone bassinet, and those allocated to have the infant sleep in the mother's bed also breastfed more frequently than those allocated the stand-alone. There was not a statistical difference between side-car or maternal bed allocation and breastfeeding frequency. Tully and Ball (2012) found that among dyads who underwent non-labor cesarean section delivery, there was a trend for more frequent breastfeeding in the group allocated the side-car compared to the group with the stand-alone bassinet, but the difference was not statistically significant. Maternal-infant sleep and midwife presence during the observation period did not vary by randomized rooming-in arrangement in either study.

The median breastfeeding frequency per observed hour and range of breastfeeding sessions were greater during the second postpartum night across conditions in the vaginal study (stand-alone 0.5 (0.0-6.6); side-car 1.3 (0.0-7.3)) than in the cesarean study (stand-alone 0.4 (0.0-1.1); side-car 0.6 (0.1-1.6)).

None of the infants experienced an adverse event during the course of either the vaginal or cesarean bassinet study. However, the height and angle of the stand-alone bassinet relative to the mother introduced several potential risks to infants. Observed stand-alone bassinet risks involved lifting infants without support for their heads, tipping the bassinet while attempting to return an infant, dropping an infant into the bassinet, infants positioned on a pillow in bed when the mother was asleep, and airway covering during swaddling.

Women enumerated advantages and disadvantages to both bassinet types, but they advocated for universal provision of the postnatal ward side-car instead of the stand-alone bassinet. Visual and physical access to infants, emotional closeness, less need for midwifery assistance, and breastfeeding facilitation were all spontaneously mentioned as side-car bassinet benefits. Tully and Ball (2012) reported that:

participants who received the stand-alone bassinet spontaneously offered that the intervention "would have made a huge difference." Most of women who had cesarean sections (29 of 35) reported that the bassinet type affected their interactions with their infants. No mother commented unfavorably on the side-car, whereas 11 of 15 (73%) stand-alone cesarean participants commented unfavorably about their allocated bassinet (p. 498).

Discussion

Our observational and qualitative findings suggest that the side-car bassinet facilitates postnatal-unit breastfeeding, and may be the most appropriate rooming-in arrangement following vaginal or cesarean childbirth. Stand-alone bassinets present an unnecessary breastfeeding obstacle. Further, the widespread rooming-in arrangement of stand-alone bassinets may pose a hazard for infants because of (a) mothers' compromised mobility during the early postpartum period after cesarean section and (b) limited maternal-infant visibility because of the bassinet design.

In both of our studies, the proportion of the observation period in which participants were awake did not vary by allocated rooming-in arrangement, so the breastfeeding associations do not reflect differential sleep amounts. That the maternal bed or side-car bassinet led to more frequent breastfeeding sessions on the postnatal unit after vaginal birth compared to those allocated the regular stand-alone bassinet suggests that some of the breastfeeding obstacles currently encountered are iatrogenic consequence of the physical separation of mothers and infants (Ball, 2008). Odent (2003) similarly states that a priority for maternity care should be "not to get in their way" (p. 80).

The limited power of the studies, related to their sample size, means that the observed differences in breastfeeding frequency may not be robust. However, the qualitative findings reflect mothers' strong preference for the side-car bassinet, including as a means to facilitate postnatal unit breastfeeding. The difference in the breastfeeding frequency results found between our two studies is most likely due to a combination of mothers experiencing greater obstacles and perceiving a lower degree of infant interest in breastfeeding after cesarean compared to following vaginal childbirth. Tully and Ball (2012) summarized that the side-car led to "easier" breastfeeding sessions among cesarean mothers, which may be vital in promoting maternal recovery in the early postpartum period.

Conclusions

Women preferred the side-car bassinet when rooming-in on the postnatal unit. Overnight filmed breastfeeding frequency significantly varied after vaginal birth, but not after cesarean section, by allocated bassinet type. More infant risks were observed with stand-alone bassinet use in both trials.

Following either vaginal or cesarean birth, stand-alone bassinets may present an unnecessary breastfeeding obstacle when rooming-in and pose a hazard for infants. Considering the needs of breastfeeding dyads may be key in facilitating more effective support. Mothers desired the standard postnatal unit environment to be more accommodating. If women continue to be offered only the stand-alone bassinet for rooming-in, then caution to mothers regarding the possibility of breastfeeding difficulty and sub-optimal infant handling may be warranted.

Acknowledgements

This research was funded by Babes-in-Arms and the Owen F. Aldis Fund. The funding sources approved of the study designs, but were not involved in data collection, analyses, writing, or publication. Kristin P. Tully is currently supported by the National Institutes of Child Health and Human Developmental Training Grant, 5T32HD007376-22.

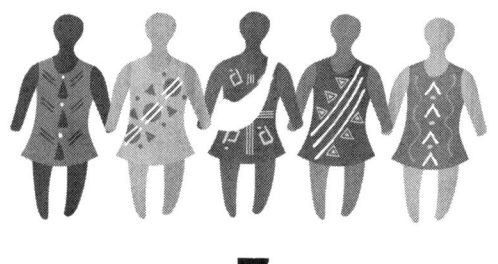

7

Increasing Access to Human Milk

Increasing the Use of Donor Human Milk: An Assessment of Knowledge, Beliefs, and Practices Among Key Stakeholders in North Carolina

Jessye Brick, Talene Ghazarian, and Taylor Marie Snyder

Background

The World Health Organization (WHO) recognizes that breastfeeding provides optimal nutrition for most infants, and therefore recommends exclusively breastfeeding for the first six months of life. Use of infant formula is associated with an increased risk of many negative health outcomes, including Sudden Infant Death Syndrome (SIDS), obesity, and asthma (U.S. Department of Health and Human Services, 2011). Yet for some mothers, breastfeeding is not an option. For these women, the WHO recommends donor human milk as the next best option (World Health Organization, 2011). In North America, there are 13 milk banks accredited by the Human Milk Banking Association of North America (HMBANA, 2012). These banks collect donations, pasteurize the milk, and distribute donor human milk to over 271 cities (HMBANA, 2013).

Donor human milk is primarily consumed by infants in Neonatal Intensive Care Units (NICUs). When infants are born prematurely, it is common for their mother's milk not to have come in at the time of their birth. Yet these infants potentially have the most to gain from consuming breast milk. Compared to premature infants who are fed infant formula, those who are given breast milk have fewer cases of sepsis and necrotizing enterocolitis (NEC), both of which are life threatening and expensive to treat. Human milk also assists with development of the gastrointestinal biome and is associated with improved cognitive skills and neurodevelopment (Cohen, 2007; Lucas & Cole, 1990).

Despite the immense health benefits of breast milk, there remains widespread ignorance of donor human milk banking and access to donor milk is problematic. In 2010, 11 states had no access to donor human milk (HMBANA, 2013). Neonatologists play a crucial role in promoting donor human milk. They drive the demand side by prescribing donor human milk to infants as well as the supply side by encouraging mothers to donate unneeded or surplus breast milk.

Method

The present study surveyed neonatologists and interviewed other key stakeholders in North Carolina in order to gain a stronger understanding of their beliefs, attitudes, and practices regarding donor human milk. The results point to directions that researchers, advocates, and policy makers can take to increase awareness, acceptability, and accessibility of donor human milk. Twelve neonatologists completed the online survey. In addition, four key informant interviews were conducted with professionals invested in milk banking: a neonatologist, a nurse manager, a nurse who works at the WakeMed Mothers' Milk Bank in Raleigh, North Carolina, and a state breastfeeding coordinator.

Results

Research findings indicated that there are several barriers to implementing widespread use of donor human milk. One such barrier is the low supply, which makes it difficult to promote donor human milk. A neonatologist said:

We seem to have just enough milk to cover our requests, so it's sort of hard to go out there and try and open up

It Takes a Village

> the world. So we don't do any marketing. It's all word of mouth.

The misperception among hospitals and health care providers of the high cost of donor human milk was another barrier identified by key informants.

> *There is a perception that it's very costly because we charge about $5/ounce ... I calculated at one point, our average very low birth weight [infant] ... was using something like 40 ounces of donor milk for their whole hospitalization ... $200 over a while hospitalization is nothing.*

Other barriers identified through key informant interviews included a lengthy donor approval process and stringent pasteurization and storage regulations. When neonatologists were asked about barriers preventing women from donating milk in the online survey, the most common answers were lack of knowledge about donor milk banks, the time involved in donation, and lack of encouragement to donate milk.

The online survey identified various approaches to increase the use of donor human milk, as outlined in Figure 1. When neonatologists were asked what strategies they believed would increase clinicians' recommendation that mothers donate their milk, the most common answers were improving the feasibility of the donation process and having an in-hospital donor milk bank.

Increasing Access to Human Milk

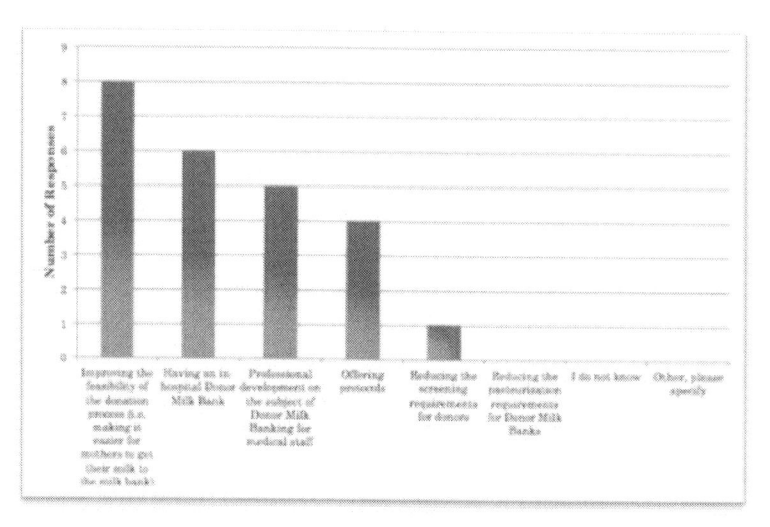

Figure 1 - *What strategies do you believe would increase clinicians' recommendations that mothers donate their milk?*

Discussion

In response to these findings, several recommendations for researchers and advocates were developed. It was recommended that researchers should investigate alternative pasteurization methods that preserve the safety, nutritional, and immunological components of breast milk, while reducing costs and staff time. The current pasteurization process, the Holder Method of pasteurization, requires that the milk be gently heated in a shaking water bath. This process retains the majority of milk's beneficial components while eliminating bacteria. Milk samples are checked for their potential contamination prior to being frozen in small batches for distribution. The complex process requires a pasteurization team, making it time consuming and expensive (HMBANA, 2013). Thus, there is a need for research on developing other techniques or modifications that reduce processing costs.

One key informant suggested that advocates could increase awareness and supply by developing a pamphlet for new mothers that uses simple language to describe the uses of donor human milk, reasons for donating, and how to donate. This pamphlet could be available in both English and Spanish and distributed in a variety of ways, including through WIC staff and health care professionals. Thus, advocates can help increase supply by both educating health care providers about the process and opportunities for donating human milk, education which would be supported by more donor milk banks.

Half of survey respondents, and various key informants, stated that having an in-hospital donor milk bank would facilitate increased use. Currently, donor milk banks cover transportation costs while requiring donors to collect, freeze, and mail a minimum of 100 ounces of breast milk at a time. Having an in-hospital milk bank would cut transportation costs, leading to a significant drop in cost of the donor milk. Hospitals might also choose to remove volume requirements for donation, making it more feasible for women to donate any amount of milk. In addition, key informants suggested that having an in-hospital milk bank would increase awareness, thus driving up both supply and demand.

The United States further stands to benefit from considering how other countries approach donor milk banking. For instance, Brazil has implemented the *Breastfeeding-Friendly Postman Program*, through which 6,000 mail carriers and firefighters have been trained to collect and transport donations of human milk. This program has greatly facilitated the donation process. The extensive network of over 150 donor milk banks provided milk for about 300,000 pre-term infants in 1999 (Dunn, 2012). Brazil is an excellent example of how the government has widely and publicly supported donor human milk banking. Such support increases awareness and normalizes both breastfeeding and the use of donor human milk.

Conclusion

The Surgeon General's Call to Action to Support Breastfeeding, released in 2011, emphasizes the need to "identify and address obstacles to greater availability of safe banked donor milk for fragile infants" (U.S. Department of Health and Human Services, 2011). Research on human milk should be expanded to assess the attitudes of neonatologists outside of North Carolina in order to gain information on the current situation in the United States. Future research should include a more representative sample of neonatologists, as well as other stakeholders, such as nurses, lactation consultants, and new parents.

It Takes a Village

The Gift of Milk: How Altruistic Milk Sharing Practices Empower Women

Aunchalee Palmquist

"Milk sharing" is an emergent infant feeding practice in which a breastfeeding mother nourishes a child who is not her own biological offspring, through privately negotiated altruistic breast milk gifts. Milk sharing via private arrangement is often called *informal, casual,* or *peer-to-peer* milk sharing, which are terms that distinguish it from breast milk donations that are processed and distributed by a human milk bank (Akre, Gribble, & Minchin, 2011; Geraghty, Heier, & Rasmussen, 2011; Gribble & Hausman, 2012). Altruistic milk sharing is distinct from milk selling, which involves marketing breast milk for profit. While milk sharing and other forms of cooperative breastfeeding (e.g., wet nursing, cross-nursing, co-nursing) and have always existed in the U.S., percolating just beneath the surface of mainstream social consciousness, it was the use of online social networking sites that catapulted milk sharing into the public gaze, transforming it into a bona fide social phenomenon.

Today, with the aid of breastfeeding technology, and the Internet, parents who desire to feed their babies human breast milk, but are unable to produce it themselves, can turn to online milk sharing networks. Unlike donor milk available through milk banks, breast milk acquired over the Internet does not require a doctor's prescription, medical eligibility, or even money; it flows freely between donors and recipients. At the same time, breast milk procured via the Internet is not screened for disease or contamination in any standard way, and is not pasteurized. Health authorities in the U.S., France, and Canada have issued formal statements warning against milk sharing due to risk of infectious diseases (Gribble & Hausman, 2012). Others caution against procuring breast milk from strangers online due to risk of microbial contamination (Keim et al., 2013). Such warnings have done little to slow the growth of Internet-facilitated milk sharing. Two sites in particular, *Eats on Feets* (EOF) and *Human Milk 4 Human Babies* (HM4HB) host two of the largest online altruistic milk sharing sites on the Internet.

The purpose of this paper is to look, for a moment, past the controversies of milk-sharing risks, and to gain perspective on the meanings and significance the practice. This examination is narrowly focused on the ways breast milk gifts symbolize generosity, empowerment, and mutual understanding among donors and recipients (Shaw & Bartlett, 2010). It is based on analyses of content shared on *Eats and Feets* (EOF) and *Human Milk 4 Human Babies* (HM4HB) Facebook sites from April 2011 through March 2013.

Analyses

A total of 1,249 posts were archived and categorized during this timeframe. Analysis of the posts followed a two-step process, the first a categorical analysis and the second a thematic analysis. Categories included requests for milk, notifications of milk to donate, general breastfeeding support and information, and links to news articles, blogs, and other media. Themes reflected content on the variety of reasons for donation, reasons for requesting breast milk, milk sharing philosophies and ideologies, discourses of milk sharing in the popular media, testimonials about the positive experiences of milk sharing, resources for breastfeeding, and information on the various strategies for collecting, storing, and delivering breast milk. Three salient themes emerged from the analyses that give insight to the meaning and significance of milk sharing practices: altruistic ideologies, empowerment, and social justice. Selected illustrative quotes drawn from the archived posts are presented verbatim.

Altruistic Milk Sharing

Altruistic giving is a guiding principle of milk sharing on EOF and HM4B sites. Altruistic milk sharing is tied up with idealized conceptualizations of breast milk as something that one cannot easily put a price tag on, something that transcends individualism and individual profit, and should be made available to every baby in need:

> *To me, milk-sharing is a political act, and a spiritual one. It says: no child is more precious than another, and all children deserve the food that is designed for them. It says, we may have different stories, different customs, different breasts, but we are all mothers to our children. It says that together, we have the power to feed our children what*

they need, and we will not be deceived, scared, placated or undermined into thinking or acting otherwise.

Donors and recipients emphasize the role of altruism in providing a safety mechanism against harm. Selling breast milk is actively discouraged, both by site administrators and members of EOF and HM4HB communities. Altruistic models of donation are theoretically safer than for-profit models, which have been associated with questionable storage, handling, and delivery practices, and potentially harmful bacterial contamination (Geraghty et al., 2013; Keim et al., 2013). Milk sharing participants also note the intrinsic safety mechanisms in altruistic models of donation:

> *I would be much more concerned with the safety of milk that's been PURCHASED and not donated! When people are making money off milk, there's more incentive to do things like dilute milk (to make it look like more) or withhold information that could turn a family off from buying (like taking potentially harmful drugs).*

Removing moneymaking incentives also eliminates economic barriers to accessing donor breast milk.

Empowerment

Empowerment through milk sharing occurs when donors and recipients exercise agency in making informed decisions about what to do with their bodies and how to care for their babies. Donors express feeling *rewarded, fulfilled,* and *grateful* for the opportunity to help other babies, particularly when they are able to see for themselves that a *milk baby is thriving* (Gribble, 2013). For example:

> *I have donated to three ladies, one of them I donated to regularly and we became friends. I met her baby girl the first time I donated to her, and it really put it in perspective for me what I was doing, and she gave me a card signed with her daughter's name and it said "thank you for helping me grow!" Made me cry! I donated roughly 1,000 ounces all together, and it was a great experience. I was extremely happy and blessed to have an oversupply and able to donate.*

Likewise, recipients express feeling empowered through milk sharing because it has provided an unexpected opportunity to nourish their baby with breast milk instead of formula. Many recipients are concerned about feeding their child infant formula, an issue that is not widely recognized, particularly in societies where formula-feeding is the social norm (Gribble & Hausman, 2012). For those individuals who have experienced breastfeeding difficulties, or who are otherwise not able to lactate, milk sharing is especially empowering:

> *I have mammary hypoplasia / IGT and am physically incapable of producing the amount of milk an infant requires. My daughters are 4 and 18 months now, and the younger daughter has had breast milk for every day of her life (aside from about two days when we ran out). She has*

received milk from nearly 50 donors, and the generosity of these women has been nothing short of profound. I have made a couple very dear friends who I otherwise would not know. Milk-sharing has opened my heart to trust. It has been a difficult road for me, with all the grieving I did about my IGT and having to swallow my sadness and put all of that aside to seek out donor milk for my daughter, to give her what was best for her. I will never forget what these women have given to our family.

Although, donors may have more leverage in milk sharing exchanges because they supply the breast milk, online posts suggest that both donors and recipients find empowerment through milk sharing.

Principals of informed choice that guide altruistic milk sharing practices are meant to empower parents, particularly those who are facing various pressures to formula-feed against their wishes, or who are dealing with social stigma related to milk sharing. HM4HB defines informed choice as:

> a choice made by competent individuals, free from coercion, that takes into account sufficient information to make a decision. This information should include benefits and risks of a course of action, as well as taking into account what alternatives are available, and an individual's intuitive feelings on the subject.

EOF describes informed choice a decision "made by examining all credible, verifiable and relevant information available, and using it to objectively weigh options as well as potential consequences." Informed milk sharing is an act of resistance against criticism that milk sharing is haphazard, unsafe, and unnecessarily places babies in harm's way.

Informed choice empowers all parents, but especially mothers, to confidently make choices that may be unconventional, but that align with their own desires, values, and beliefs about what is best for their child. The empowerment that women experience through milk sharing is most pronounced in posts that describe going against a health care provider's recommendation to formula-feed, deciding instead to milk share with positive, measureable health outcomes for the baby. Shared breast milk is often called *lifesaving, liquid gold,* and *a miracle.*

Social Justice

Social justice is promoted as a core value of milk sharing sites. Altruism, empowerment, and social justice are inextricably linked in online milk sharing discourses. As a social movement, milk sharing is described as an act that transcends individuals. Milk sharing promotes access to anyone who wants or needs it, from sick infants, to healthy babies, older children, adoptive parents, and to children and adults facing chronic diseases. It promotes the idea that breastfeeding is a basic human right, which can be realized by removing economic and social barriers to donor breast milk. Milk-sharing communities also actively work to normalize milk sharing by circulating images of milk sharing, organizing community milk-sharing events, and engaging members of online communities to share their experiences with one another.

Conclusion

Milk sharing empowers parents through principals of altruistic giving and informed choice, both of which enhance personal agency. It is actively pursued as a form of resistance to medicalization of infant feeding and third-party regulation of breast milk. Empowerment through milk sharing is multi-dimensional and occurs in varying ways depending on the individuals involved and the contexts in which it occurs. Milk sharing is also a social justice movement, casting the ability for an infant to receive breast milk as a basic human right and opening multiple channels for the flow of breast milk to reach babies in need.

Donor Human Milk: Past, Present and Future

Emily C. Taylor, Kathy Parry, and Miriam H. Labbok

Human milk should be regarded as the normative infant feeding substance as formula is associated with significant risk for acute and chronic diseases. These risks are applicable to all infants, and are also especially hazardous for preterm infants who are most vulnerable (AAP, 1997; Ip et al., 2007; Tully, 2002). As modern technologies enable the survival of babies at earlier and earlier gestational ages, there is a need and responsibility to optimize their outcomes in life. And one critical mechanism is provision of human milk. However, having not experienced the physiologic and hormonal changes of a full-term gestation, mothers of preterm infants typically require additional support to begin producing milk and to build and maintain adequate supply to meet the needs of their delicate newborn (Geddes, 2013; Montagne et al., 1999). If mother's own milk is not available, donor milk is the recommended substitute (AAP, 1997; Underwood, 2013).

When the W.K. Kellogg Foundation (WKKF) began to develop its "First Food Movement," a collective impact funding strategy to improve support for breastfeeding in the United States, it was apparent that donor milk banking is widely accepted as a critical strategy for decreasing infant mortality. However, there is little in the way of systematic review regarding the current practice in the United States. In order to inform efforts to improve donor milk banking and/or access to donor milk, WKKF commissioned the Carolina Global Breastfeeding Institute to conduct a comprehensive external assessment. This paper presents some early findings of the assessment.

Past

Early medical texts, artwork from ancient Greece and Egypt, and other historical documents suggest that women have always shared milk. The earliest available literary reference is from the 2nd century, from a physician named Soranus of Ephesus, who warned that a mother's milk was no good for the first 20 days after giving birth. Accordingly, in Ancient Greece, those who could afford it hired special slaves called *doulos* as wet nurses. Soranus promoted the use of slaves between the ages of 20-40, and recommended that they be self-controlled, good-tempered, of good color, tidy, and Greek. There is evidence to suggest that women living in the 13th century made more money working as wet nurses than any other occupation available to women (Baumslag, 1995).

Early in the twentieth century, the belief in disease transfer via microbes began to proliferate. Some physician's hypothesized that human milk may be a vehicle for disease transmission, and documented incidence of wet nursing decreased. Around this time, medical and social texts start to include discussion of the potential merits of artificial baby milk, especially in texts regarding how to feed infants whose mothers were unable to provide their own milk. The early artificial feeding products commonly resulted in infant death, most likely due to inadequate sterilization and hygiene practices. In the mid-19th century, there was an increased medicalization of childbirth and infant care, and physician and mothers' roles were shifting more generally. By the 1950s, most hospitals and health professionals promoted artificial feeding as the best feeding method, despite the established correlation between infant formulas and infant mortality (Baumslag, 1995).

It Takes a Village

Those concerned about the correlation between infant formula and mortality continued to explore how human milk could be provided to those at the highest risk of sickness and death. In 1919, the first American milk bank opened at the Boston Floating Children's Hospital. The milk bank collected and distributed unprocessed milk to ill and premature infants, and reported positive results in babies whose survival was unexpected. Donors were paid for their milk, and recipients were charged between $0.10 and $0.30 per ounce (Jones, 2003). Donors would express between 15 and 72 ounces per day, and only 40 donors were approved (compare this to current practice, where donors typically express 4-10 ounces/day for the milk bank, and HMBANA milk banks approved 3,000+ donors in 2011). This marked the first time in history that any human bodily product was sold or shared in a disembodied form (meaning not communicated directly from donor to recipient, as in wet nursing or early blood transfusion procedures; Swanson, 2011).

In the 1950s, the expectation for highly medicalized processes led to the development of guidelines for formal donor human milk banking. As milk bankers of the day adopted more and more of the blood banking model (being developed as part of the war effort), they stopped paying donors for their milk, and instead offered informal incentives, like clothing swaps (Swanson, 2011). By the 1980s, an estimated 30 milk banks were operational in the United States (Jones, 2003). And in 1985, the Human Milk Banking Association of North America was established primarily to establish standards for all North American milk banks. HMBANA collaborated with the United States Food and Drug Administration, the Centers for Disease Control and Prevention, and the American Academy of Pediatrics to develop guidelines for collection, processing, and distribution of donor human milk, published in 1990 (HMBANA, 1990).

Guidelines and recommendations for donor milk banking became more and more stringent as the HIV/AIDS epidemic spread across the globe. Many milk banks closed, though it is unknown whether they closed due to fear of spreading the disease through milk (at a time when it was still unknown what the disease was, let alone how it spread), actual or anticipated decrease in demand, or other reasons (Jones, 2003).

Present

At present, there are non-profit milk banks (associated with Human Milk Banking Association of North America), and for-profit milk banks (associated with Prolacta Bioscience, Inc.). HMBANA milk banks include 13 fully-operational, three developing (organizations in the advanced planning stages), one mentoring (organizations in the early planning stages), and 156 milk depots (designated sites which collect donated milk to be processed and distributed by an affiliate milk bank; HMBANA, 2014). Almost all milk donated to HMBANA is pasteurized and distributed as pasteurized donor human milk for those with a prescription

It Takes a Village

– mostly infants in the NICU. HMBANA remains the only professional organization for milk banking professionals, and member organization for non-profit milk banks in the United States.

Prolacta donors select from twelve choices of milk banks. All milk banks are operated solely for recruitment. No milk bank partnered or affiliated with Prolacta qualifies donors or collects, tests, or processes milk. All milk donations are sent directly to Prolacta headquarters for processing and distribution. (In this way, Prolacta milk banks are fundamentally different than the traditional definition of "milk banks" in the U.S.) Until 2013, all milk donated to Prolacta was processed into nutritional products for preterm infants in Neonatal Intensive Care Units (NICUs), except for a portion of the milk donated to the "International Breast Milk Project," which is tested, pasteurized, standardized, and shipped to Africa for infants who do not have safe access to their own mother's milk. They produced four fortifiers, each intended to achieve particular caloric counts when added to the mother's own milk, and one specifically for trophic feeds. In August of 2013, Prolacta launched three new products: Prolact HMTM, Prolact CRTM and Prolact RTFHM (Ready to Feed), all standardized, pasteurized donor human milk for use alone or with mother's milk (Prolacta Bioscience, 2014).

In 2010, the FDA Pediatric Advisory Committee (FDA 2011) convened a meeting to "obtain a better understanding of current practices, infectious disease risk, state regulations, and mitigation strategies currently used to avoid contamination of donated milk." The FDA PAC heard from experts in the field, including HMBANA and Prolacta affiliates, unaffiliated researchers on the topic, and members of the public. The meeting had four major themes. The first theme was an endorsement of human milk banking by the Pediatric Therapeutics Committee of the FDA.

The second theme was a concern about Internet and person-to-person milk exchange, which the FDA strongly discourages. The third theme was the need to address currently inconsistent and lacking state regulations for donor human milk in order to attend to "illegitimate milk banking operations" (though it was acknowledged that HMBANA and Prolacta processing appropriately mitigate risk; FDA, 2011). And the fourth was the need for greater and more transparent monitoring and evaluation. There was consensus that there is a need for further research on the risks and benefits of pasteurized donor human milk, human and cow's milk fortifiers, and exclusive versus supplemental feedings. The FDA encouraged HMBANA and Prolacta to create a registry to generate an outcome profile for recipients of donor human milk (and related products; ADA, 2011; FDA, 2010).

In the three years subsequent to this meeting, the FDA Working Group on Infant Formula has continued to explore the field in an effort to determine appropriate regulation and inspection of banked donor milk. According to one milk bank affiliate:

> *They're just not caught up ... FDA regulation would give us clout with the insurance companies ... Without regulation, the insurance companies are not willing to pay attention to us and that's a crime, really. I think informed regulation is the ideal to bring donor human milk to all vulnerable babies who need it.*

Milk sharing, having been practiced since the beginning of human history, has recently been the subject of intense public and clinical debate. According to *Human Milk 4 Human Babies Informed Milk Sharing Network* (HM4HB), "milk sharing is a vital tradition that has been taken from us, and it is crucial that we regain trust in ourselves, our neighbors, and in our fellow women." In contrast:

> The FDA recommends that if, after consultation with a health care provider, you decide to feed a baby with human milk from a source other than the baby's mother, you should only use milk from a source that has screened its milk donors and taken other precautions to ensure the safety of its milk (FDA 2010).

Despite the (seemingly growing) fervor of the debate, milk sharing happens every day in the United States.

As public knowledge about the importance of breastfeeding increased, so too has the buying and selling of human milk. At present, all laws regulating the sale of products dependent on donation from a human (living or deceased) exclude human milk, much like other "replenishable" products, such as sperm or hair. As such, there is very little information available to characterize the practice. In this assessment, milk bank donors and affiliates, and physicians reported a general negative perception of selling milk in key informant interviews. This negative perception resonates with three themes: the potential for corruption, an ethically gray area, and the fear of selling being a scam. The potential for corruption and the ethically gray aspects of milk selling both highlight the problem of mothers donating for the wrong reasons.

Content analyses of milk selling sites reveal an emphasis on community, empowerment, relationships, fairness, and sisterhood. Like HM4HB, the most popular site for buying and selling milk was started by a "mom who wants the best for [her] baby" who created a place for other moms like her "to connect." *Onlythebreast.com* features a section entitled, "Moms Cry Out," where quotes from women looking to sell their milk abound. Representative of many quotes on the site, "milkmommy" says:

> *I completely agree with all of you. I'm a healthy 28 yr. old w/ a thriving 9-month-old daughter and an abundance of milk in my freezer. I don't smoke, drink, or do drugs. It is absurd to me that mothers who spend large amounts of their days pumping extra milk can't be compensated, while the milk banks are making millions!!*

Future

The final findings, analysis and recommendations are available from the Carolina Global Breastfeeding Institute online at *http://cgbi.sph.unc.edu/what-we-do/programs-and-initiatives/toolkits/donor-milk.*

8

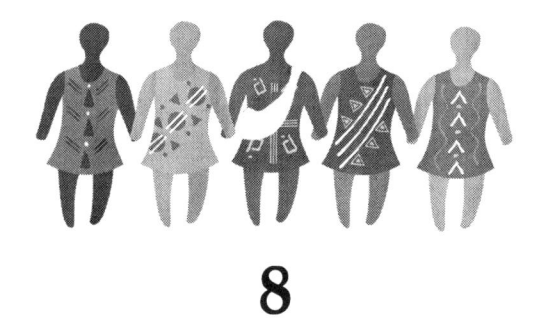

Expanding and Improving Media Support for Breastfeeding

Chasing the Numbers: Measuring Social Influences on Breastfeeding

Sheryl W. Abrahams

Purpose and Objectives

It takes a community to support breastfeeding. But how does one actually define and measure influences on breastfeeding at the community level? Behavioral theory provides an evidence-based framework for understanding social influences on breastfeeding, as well as for designing and evaluating breastfeeding promotion interventions (Glanz, Rimer, & Viswanath, 2008; Khoury, Moazzem, Jarjoura, Carothers, & Hinton, 2005; Kloeblen, Thompson, & Miner, 1999; Kools, Thijs, & de Vries, 2005; Manstead, Proffitt, & Smart, 1983; Sittlington, Stewart-Knox, Wright, Bradbury, & Scott, 2007; Williams, Innis, Vogel, & Stephen, 1999). A theory-driven approach to breastfeeding promotion may help improve breastfeeding promotion program planning, and intervention effectiveness, and maximize the information available from program evaluations (Glanz et al., 2008).

This presentation will explore how researchers and practitioners may use theory-driven approaches to move from a general idea of community-level support, towards specific constructs that can be measured and targeted for change. Using evidence from behavioral public health, it will discuss ways to define, operationalize and measure interpersonal and community-level influences on breastfeeding, and discuss implications for breastfeeding promotion practice.

Method

Based on a non-systematic literature review, the author identified behavioral theories and models that have been tested in the context of breastfeeding initiation and continuation, and identified theory constructs shown to have good reliability and validity in capturing social influences on breastfeeding. This search included influences acting at the interpersonal level (i.e., family, friends, employers, etc.), as well as those acting at the broader community level (Khoury et al., 2005; Kloeblen et al., 1999; Kools et al., 2005; Manstead et al., 1983; Sittlington et al., 2007). The review was restricted to more direct measures of social influences on breastfeeding behaviors, as opposed to social influences on breastfeeding beliefs and attitudes.

Findings

Behavioral theories with evidence-based applications in breastfeeding promotion include the Theory of Reasoned Action (TRA) and the closely-related Theory of Planned Behavior (TPB), as well as the Transtheoretical Model (TTM), and Social Cognitive Theory (SCT) (Khoury et al., 2005; Kloeblen et al., 1999; Kools et al., 2005; Manstead et al., 1983; Sittlington et al., 2007; Williams et al., 1999). Social influences on breastfeeding can be described by several constructs derived from these and other theories, including: social norms, behavioral control, observational learning and social support (Glanz et al., 2008; Khoury et al., 2005; Kloeblen et al., 1999; Kools et al., 2005; Manstead et al., 1983; Sittlington et al., 2007; Vari, Camburn, & Henly, 2000; Williams et al., 1999).

Theory of Reasoned Action/ Theory of Planned Behavior

The TRA, and the closely-related TPB, state that a given behavior is most influenced by intentions to perform the behavior, and that those intentions are in turn determined by individual attitudes towards the behavior, perceptions of the social norms surrounding the behavior, and perceived control over the behavior (Glanz et al., 2008). Evidence indicates that the broader social environment influences breastfeeding behaviors through its effect on both subjective norms and perceived behavioral control (Khoury et al., 2005; Kloeben et al., 1999; Kools et al., 2005; Manstead et al., 1983; Sittlington et al., 2007).

Subjective norms are measured by tallying mothers' Likert-scale answers to a series of questions about whether certain significant individuals approve or disapprove of breastfeeding or formula-feeding (for example, "My spouse would approve of my breastfeeding.") (Glanz et al., 2008; Khoury et al., 2005; Kloeblen et al., 1999; Kools et al., 2005; Manstead et al., 1983; Sittlington et al., 2007). Perceived behavioral control is measured according to a semantic differential scale (for example, "Breastfeeding is ... very much under my control/ under my control/ somewhat under my control/ not under my control"; Glanz et al., 2008; Manstead et al., 1983; Kools et al., 2005; Sittlington et al., 2007).

Because both constructs rely on an individual mothers' perceptions of the broader social context, it is possible to change these perceptions without changing the actual social context itself. It is conversely possible to change the actual social context, without achieving concomitant changes in individual mothers' perceptions (Glanz et al., 2008).

Transtheoretical Model

The TTM suggests that individuals progress through different stages of change on their way to deciding whether to practice a given health behavior. Individuals who are closer to taking up a health promoting behavior will practice more processes of change including using helping relationships (seeking and using social support for the healthy behavior change; Glanz et al., 2008). Evidence supports the TTM's usefulness in predicting breastfeeding intention (Kloeblen et al., 1999). Breastfeeding peer counseling is one example of a helping relationship that provides social support for positive breastfeeding behaviors, as is building trust and rapport with health care providers supportive of breastfeeding (Kloeblen et al., 1999). Based on the TTM, individuals at further stages of change will be more amenable to establishing and using these healthy relationships, compared to individuals at preliminary stages.

Social Cognitive Theory and Social Support

Evidence supports the application of the Social Cognitive Theory to both breastfeeding initiation and duration (Williams et al., 1999). The construct of social support is central to both Social Cognitive Theory, and has also been shown to predict breastfeeding independently of a specific behavioral framework (Vari et al., 2000). Empirical and theoretical research support the existence of four types of social support: emotional support (including trust, empathy and caring), instrumental support (including tangible services), informational support, and appraisal support (constructive feedback) (Glanz et al., 2008). Because different types of individuals are best placed to offer different types of social support (unrelated individuals are traditionally the most effective sources of informational support, for example), the effectiveness of social support in breastfeeding promotion may depend on what type of support is offered by whom (Glanz et al., 2008).

Discussion and Conclusions

Operationalizing and measuring theory-based constructs that capture social influences on infant feeding, and focusing on those most predictive of breastfeeding, can help improve success as part of a theory-driven approach to community breastfeeding promotion (Glanz et al., 2008). Evidence supports the use of several different behavioral models and associated constructs in the understanding of individual breastfeeding behaviors (Khoury et al., 2005; Kloeblen et al., 1999; Kools et al., 2005; Manstead et al., 1983; Sittlington et al., 2007; Vari et al., 2000; Williams et al., 1999). These constructs include perceived social norms and perceived behavioral control as described by the TRA/ TPB, the use of helping relationships and other processes of change as described by the TTM, and social support as described by the SCT and other models (Glanz et al., 2008; Khoury et al., 2005; Kloeblen et al., 1999; Kools et al, 2005; Manstead et al, 1983; Sittlington et al., 2007; Vari et al., 2000; Williams et al., 1999). Public health practitioners who are designing and evaluating breastfeeding promotion programs would do well to make use of these and other evidence-based constructs, as well as of established best practices for their operationalization and measurement.

Implications for the applicability of the concepts of perceived social norms and behavioral control include the fact that promotion programs that seek to change existing social norms and influences on breastfeeding must also be sure to change mothers' perceptions of these norms and influences. At the same time, breastfeeding promotion programs may be able to achieve successes through changing individual mothers' perceptions of their social environment, regardless of whether they effect any changes on the environment itself. The applicability of the TTM to breastfeeding behaviors further indicates that the use of peer counselors, and the fostering of other helpful relationships, may be most effective if targeted to individuals in more advanced stages of change. Given the importance of social support to breastfeeding promotion efforts, public health practitioners must differentiate between types of social support, and recognize which types of individuals are best placed to provide the necessary support.

Future research is needed to identify additional theories and models of behavior change that are predictive of breastfeeding behaviors, as well as to evaluate behavioral models as they apply to breastfeeding support by health care providers, employers, and others.

It Takes a Village

Mediating Mother Support: Social Networks, Online Discussion, and Breastfeeding Support

Emily B. Anzicek

As the popularity and prevalence of computer mediated communication (CMC) and social networks continue to increase, so does the use of these forms of communication to offer support for people facing a range of issues across the lifespan. Breastfeeding is one of those issues. However, very little research exists specifically about online breastfeeding support. This study examines the use of CMC to provide breastfeeding support via discussion boards and Facebook groups. While CMC has democratized access to support groups and communities, a number of problems and challenges exist, especially when the support groups are for breastfeeding mothers.

Background

The drastic difference between the recommendations of the medical community and the length of time most infants in the U.S. are breastfed begs the question as to why mothers stop breastfeeding prior to the recommended amount of time. The answer to this is multifaceted and complicated. One major barrier to breastfeeding identified by *The Surgeon General's Call to Action* in 2011 is "poor family and social support" (p. 12). According to *The Call to Action* (2011), "Women with friends who have breastfed successfully are more likely to choose to breastfeed. On the other hand, negative attitudes of family and friends can pose a barrier to breastfeeding" (p. 12). *The Call to Action* (2011) notes, "Some mothers say that they do not ask for help with breastfeeding from their family or friends because of the contradictory information they receive from these sources" (p. 12). Since lack of support is such a serious barrier to successful breastfeeding, clearly alternative sources of support are necessary and vital.

One such alternative source is online support groups. Mothers frequently use the Internet to seek information about all sorts of child- and parenting-related issues. In their 2009 study of parental information-seeking, Plantin and Daneback (2009) cite a market study by Yahoo! that estimated that 86% of parents used the Internet to search for information (p. 2). Increasingly, support groups are part of that information-seeking process. According to Plantin and Daneback (2009), "the generally accepted reason for this is the postmodern circumstances of parenthood that put increasingly risk-aware parents without support from their immediate friends and family" (p. 3). However, the authors found that a great deal of misleading, unusable, and even dangerous information exists on websites targeted at parents, and that determining the source and veracity of the information can be confusing and difficult for parents seeking answers about health-related topics (Plantin & Daneback, 2009, p. 7). As noted in *The Surgeon General's Call to Action*, incorrect and inconsistent information can have a chilling effect on the breastfeeding mother's support seeking.

It Takes a Village

While inaccurate and dangerous information is a major concern in online support groups, Barak et al. (2008) note that support groups have long existed and developed from the idea that "people who share similar difficulties, misery, pain, disease, condition, or distress may both understand one another better than those who do not and offer mutual emotional and pragmatic support" (p. 1868). Further, the authors argue that participation in online support groups provide participants with a sense of empowerment ("the ability to make personal decisions, exercise critical thinking, and to access relevant resources") over their situation that would not be possible with therapy, counseling, or professional care alone (Barak et al., 2008, p. 1868). Barak et al. (2008) argue that the major benefits of online support groups come from the fact that people tend to be less interpersonally inhibited in CMC and because the act of writing (which tends to be the mode of communication in online support groups) is emotionally cathartic (pp. 1870, 1872).

Like Plantin and Daneback (2009), though Barak et al. (2008) see potential problems with online support groups. Since many, if not most, of these groups are not moderated by professionals or experts in the topics they address, it is not uncommon for online support groups to develop "maladaptive belief systems" based on incorrect or incomplete interpretations of scientific research and hostility toward the authorities of clinicians and experts (Barak et. al, 2008, p. 1878). Clearly, this has implications for online breastfeeding support since these maladaptive belief systems can cause problems for mothers that can lead to early weaning.

Methodology

For this study, four online breastfeeding support groups were examined, three in the form of discussion forums hosted on websites and two in the form of Facebook group pages. These groups differ in how they are facilitated, who owns them, to whom the groups are open, and the speed at which conversations happened. From each group, I took posts from 48 consecutive hours. On those posts, I performed a close reading and textual analysis to look for themes about breastfeeding, supportive and unsupportive communication, and influences of outside sources. I did not participate in any of the conversations that occurred on any of the groups. The selected groups are: the breastfeeding discussion forum on *BabyCenter.com*, *LLLI.org* (La Leche League International)'s discussion forums, *Kellymom.com*'s Facebook breastfeeding support group, and a local Facebook breastfeeding support group from a major Midwestern university town.

Results

The facilitation of discussions, quality of information, and level of supportiveness differed drastically among the observed groups. Of the four groups, BabyCenter's support forum was the only one not facilitated by an expert or professional leader. As such, the quality of information shared by the group members was the lowest of the four communities, with potentially damaging and even incorrect information shared among the members. Furthermore, advertising from bottle manufacturers, pacifier manufacturers, and vitamin supplement manufacturers appeared on BabyCenter's support forum pages. These advertisements were from non-WHO Code compliant companies, such as brands that advertise bottles and pacifiers to the public, so images of bottles and pacifiers frequently appeared alongside of breastfeeding advice and support. La Leche League's forums, facilitated by La Leche League employees and leaders, offered evidence-based support to participants, but tended toward the clinical at times in how that support was communicated. No advertising appeared on any La Leche League forum page.

The two Facebook groups offered their own challenges and benefits, in many ways different from the discussion boards. Both Facebook groups are monitored by lactation professionals. However, most of the support offered came from peer participants in the groups. The Kellymom group moved incredibly quickly, making it difficult to keep up with all of the questions being asked and answered. The responses were often supported by evidence in the form of links to reputable sources of information about breastfeeding. The localized group, also quite busy and fast-moving, tended to offer more emotional support and frequently veers away from the topic of breastfeeding and on to more broad parenting concerns. As is the nature of Facebook, advertising frequently appears on these group pages and owners have very little control over what advertising their users see.

Discussion

The importance of online support groups to the community of breastfeeding mothers should not be understated. These groups offer peer and sometimes even professional support, despite the boundaries of geography, time, and socioeconomic status. However, more work needs to be done to provide proper support and information to mothers who seek it online. First of all, care must be taken to ensure that mothers receive correct information when they turn to discussion boards and online communities for breastfeeding support. This can be achieved through the use of professional or expert facilitators, only accepting advertising from WHO Code-compliant marketers, and understanding the belief systems about breastfeeding that develop in these support groups.

Second, providers need to examine the effects of socioeconomic status on mothers' ability to access support online. As long as the "digital divide" is defined by socioeconomic status and demographics, access to the benefits of breastfeeding support will be unequal in the United States. Finally, newer forms of social media, like Google+ Hangouts, and Skype should be considered for use in providing breastfeeding support.

It Takes a Village

A Look at the World Breastfeeding Week Public Announcement Videos in Quebec, "*Je l'ai fait ... / I did it ...*" and "*Allaitement c'est glamour / Breastfeeding is Glamour*"

Carole Dobrich

Breastfeeding in the media is often portrayed in a negative manner, even to the degree of being called sexual. The social-media giant, Facebook, is renowned for removing breastfeeding photos from their site or blocking user access to their pages because the "content is considered offensive." The image of a baby or child at the breast needs to be normalized so no one blinks an eye when an image appears.

During World Breastfeeding Week 2012 in Montreal, Quebec, two breastfeeding videos were released. I wanted to present the reaction of both health care professionals and the public to the two breastfeeding campaign videos.

Montreal is known for celebrating World Breastfeeding Week each year, and focuses on breastfeeding in public. The 2012 Montreal Public Health Department campaign was titled, *Moi aussi j'allaite... Allaiter, c'est GLAMOUR* (I am breastfeeding too ... Breastfeeding is glamorous). The campaign played on the French wording *glamour* and *l'amour*, the word for love. The Montreal Public Health Department also offers a professional lactation education day for health care professionals during this week along with the breastfeeding in public campaign. Both videos were shown that

Expanding and Improving Media Support for Breastfeeding

day, and the breastfeeding spokeswoman and Quebec actress, Mayee Payement, also attended and shared her experience. She loved breastfeeding. She wanted mothers to know they could breastfeed anywhere, anytime, even when attending a glamorous evening event.

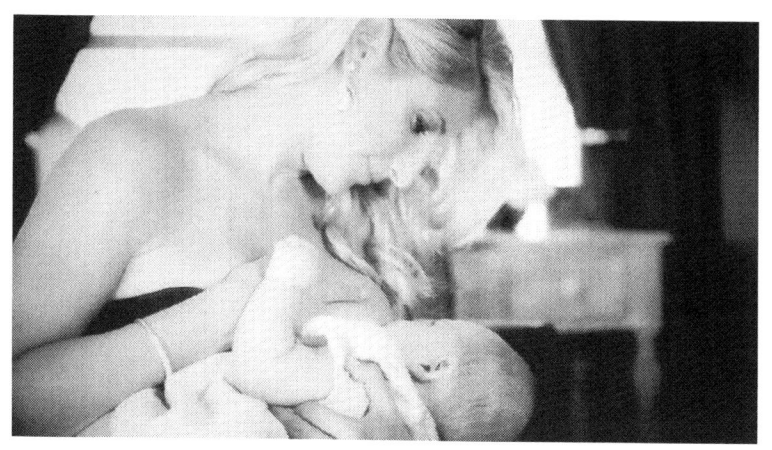

http://www.youtube.com/watch?v=WpivMPwMOGw

This breastfeeding campaign could be perceived as "sexy" and "glamorous" and Montreal is well known for that. Yet the media feasted on the campaign, *Moi aussi j'allaite... Allaiter, c'est GLAMOUR. http://www.youtube.com/watch?v=WpivMPwMOGw*, and it was not always positive. Either way, the media was talking about breastfeeding, on the news, in the newspapers, and on social media pages.

I am a supporter of the breastfeed anywhere, anytime promotion, and this, to me, was just one of those anywhere, anytime ideas. Others did not see it like that and Facebook comments from different pages varied from, *"I thought we*

It Takes a Village

had finally gotten away from the breastfeeding and sex image," and *"This is going to set breastfeeding in public back 10 years."* Others loved it as she was expressing how she felt about breastfeeding—empowered. She is an actress and a mother, and she is sexy. What is the big deal?! Just because women have babies and breastfeed doesn't mean they lose their sexuality. Yet, that is what the media seems to want to portray to the public, the maternal Madonna image. Wake up, media, you are doing the public a disservice.

I had thought for many years, how to present breastfeeding in public as normal, as something that is part of our everyday lives. Something that most women do or have done and something that is so common, it can be done anywhere. I wanted to present something that drew interest from all generations, and something that particularly interested our future generation of parents to be—our teenagers. How do we get teenagers talking about breastfeeding? You don't tell them it is about breastfeeding!

With this in mind INFACT Quebec decided to "play on this theme" and release its first video during World Breastfeeding Week 2012.

The INFACT Quebec video was made to reflect breastfeeding in public. We wanted it to interest adolescents and young adults. The script was very simple and drew on curiosity. What are teenagers curious about? Sex! *"Je l'ai fait"* ... "I did it" ... Did what you ask? There is no mention of breastfeeding in the title and the video is very simple.

Expanding and Improving Media Support for Breastfeeding

It shows the faces of different aged women saying, *"je l'ai fait dans le bain,"* or *"I did it on the kitchen counter,"* and the many places that they had breastfed. They did it in a lake, on a mountain, while camping, in a canoe, in front of their kids, just about everywhere. Only the last few images have

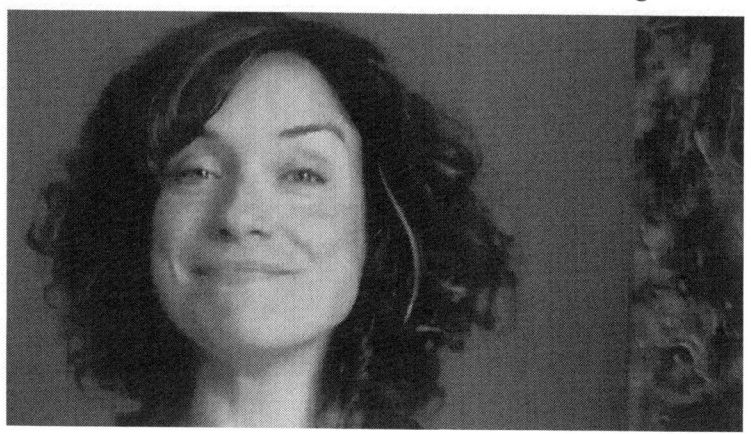

http://www.youtube.com/watch?v=Bh8XKKxpsEc .

women breastfeeding and stating *"breastfeeding anywhere, any time, it's natural."*

We had both boys and girls, aged 13 to 20, read or listen to the beginning of the script before they saw the complete video to see their reactions. They were smiling and were asking, "What are they talking about?" They all smiled and had positive comments when they saw the video. Big smiles, lots of laughter, and questions like, *"Is it really possible to have done it in all those places?"* were asked. All of the adolescents we spoke to liked the video because they saw it as a play on their curiosity about sex, yet it presented breastfeeding instead of sex in the same curious manner.

It Takes a Village

Will it increase breastfeeding rates? Who knows? It did get adolescents and young adults talking about breastfeeding, as well as others.

Both of these World Breastfeeding Week 2012 campaign videos presented women as not only breastfeeding mothers, but as women who are empowered to be proud of what they do or have done.

The YouTube *Moi aussi j'allaite... Allaiter, c'est GLAMOUR* has 28,493 views, 27 likes and 12 dislikes, so people are looking at it.

The YouTube *"Je l'ai fait"* ... "I did it" ... has 9,800 views, 57 likes 1 dislike.

The video URL appears to have reached the Facebook radar and has been blocked several times when I have tried to repost it on the INFACT Quebec Facebook page to update our members on how the video is going. This past week, a message appeared on the screen telling me that *"The content of this video has been reported as offensive,"* so I guess we have made a significant impact if it is upsetting Facebook! Please enjoy the videos and continue to share them around the world.

Portrayals and Representations of Infant Feeding Practices in Primetime U.S. Television Media: A Discourse Analysis

Camille Fabiyi and Sarah Redman

While U.S. breastfeeding rates have improved, the U.S. still lags behind other developed countries in breastfeeding outcomes. Considerable demographic variability also exists for these outcomes, in that breastfeeding rates are lowest among young women, Black women, those who have less than a college education, and those who are at or below the poverty level (Eidelman et al., 2012). The media represents one of many macro-level factors that can shape a woman's breastfeeding attitudes, intentions, and practices (Bentley, Dee, & Jensen, 2003).

Limited systematic research has been conducted on the portrayal of breastfeeding in the media (Brown & Peuchaud, 2008; Foss & Southwell, 2006; Frerichs, Andsager, Campo, Aquilino, & Dyer, 2006; Henderson, Kitzinger, & Green, 2000), especially the U.S. television media (Foss, 2012). The purpose of this study was to examine how infant feeding, particularly breastfeeding, is represented and portrayed in primetime television media in the United States among a diverse sample of mothers.

It Takes a Village

Method

Discourse analysis is a qualitative technique used to examine a "communicative event" within the context of how society uses language or "its orders of discourse." Discourse analysis examines the relationship between the three dimensions of a communicative event: the text (spoken, written non-verbal cues used to produce meaning), the discursive practices of a community (how the text is produced and consumed), and the sociocultural context of the event (the immediate situational context or the wider backdrop like the economic, political, or cultural landscape in which it exists; Fairclough, 2000). The purpose of discourse analysis is to examine a text "not only as form, meaning, and mental process, but as complex structures and hierarchies of interaction and social practice, and their functions in context, society, and culture" (van Djik, 1997).

Using an iterative and "inductive process of decontextualization and recontextualization" (Ayres, Kavanaugh, & Knafl, 2003), we used discourse analysis to distill the meaning about how breastfeeding is viewed in society as reflected in six primetime fictional television shows (*Bones, The Office, Friday Night Lights, Grey's Anatomy, Let's Stay Together,* and *Modern Family*) from two genres (comedy and drama). Each television show was considered a communicative event. This sample of television shows was selected because they feature a diverse range of characters that parent infants, and could be viewed on the Internet through Netflix and Hulu. Seven mothers were featured on these six shows. Of these mothers, three were White, two were Black, one was biracial (half-Chinese), and one was Latina. Most were married and worked outside the home.

Our analysis was guided by key concepts from two theoretical frameworks: 1) social modeling from social-cognitive theory (Bandura, 2004), and 2) sexual objectification from feminist theory (Bartky, 1990; Frederickson & Roberts, 1997). In this study we sought to understand: 1) how society views infant feeding, including breastfeeding; 2) the extent to which portrayals reflect current infant feeding recommendations; 3) who the target audience is for each show and what the portrayal conveys to them; and, 4) what messages are conveyed about who should or is breastfeeding.

Findings

Six primetime fictional television shows were examined. Four of these shows featured mothers from diverse racial/ethnic and socioeconomic backgrounds. Breastfeeding was primarily discussed or inferred by the main maternal character as opposed to depicted. Only two of the six shows actually portrayed the main maternal character breastfeeding her infant. Three cross-cutting themes were identified. In the first theme, breasts were objectified in depictions where breastfeeding or lactation were portrayed, discussed, or inferred. Across scenes from *The Office*, *Grey's Anatomy*, and *Modern Family*, we found that mothers who breastfed were empowered to do so, but were disempowered in their encounters with others, including co-workers, strangers, and husbands. Breasts were also objectified and sexualized in certain depictions.

Another theme that emerged in our analysis relates to a tension that we observed, in that breastfeeding was seen as both a hassle and was also idealized as the mark of being a "good" parent. In scenes from *Bones* and *Friday Night Lights*, we observed mothers who described breastfeeding as a task that was restrictive to their lifestyle and diet. In other scenes, from *The Office* and *Bones*, discussions about breastfeeding were idealized by mothers as if to suggest the behavior made one a real parent.

In our last theme, we found that current breastfeeding trends and practices were reflected through the discourse across the sample of television shows. Privileged mothers, particularly those who stayed at home, those with access to maternity leave, and those with job flexibility, were portrayed as having more opportunities to breastfeed their infant in *Bones, Friday Night Lights,* and *Modern Family*. In season one of *Let's Stay Together*, a show whose audience is primarily African American, we noted a virtual absence of breastfeeding or nursing. In one scene of the show, we observed both the mother and father preparing bottles of formula almost in an assembly line fashion while discussing an unrelated matter. Similarly, on *The Office*, we also found portrayals that highlight how unsupportive hospital and work environments can inhibit optimal breastfeeding behaviors. In sum, many of the portrayals reflect current demographic trends related to who is and who is not breastfeeding. The portrayals also reflected current trends in hospital and workplace practices where it has been documented that most mothers do not give birth in Baby-Friendly facilities and do not receive adequate lactation support from their employers (Centers for Disease Control and Prevention, 2010).

Discussion/Implications

Television media represents one of many venues for promoting public health messages, and it is uniquely positioned to portray breastfeeding as a normative behavior. However, we found very few instances of infant feeding, especially breastfeeding, actually portrayed in our sample. The portrayals and depictions that were observed seemed to reflect current breastfeeding trends and practices, and likely do not move towards normalizing this behavior. There were some limitations to this analysis. First, our findings are not generalizable. We also did not include a comprehensive sample of television shows in our analysis. One strength of this study is that it integrates concepts from behavioral and feminist theory. This research is also interdisciplinary, bridging public health and communication.

Media discourse is positioned to advance social change around breastfeeding norms. Bandura's (2004) concept of social modeling suggests that people learn through observing the success and mistakes of others. This concept also

It Takes a Village

applies to media discourse around breastfeeding norms. For instance, television media can include more positive breastfeeding models. Many television shows feature infants, but very few depict mothers succeeding in their attempts to breastfeed. Lastly, television media can work with the public health community to include more positive breastfeeding messages in its storylines, where messages are tailored to specific audiences and portray breastfeeding mothers as a natural part of the community and workplace (Brown & Peuchaud, 2008).

The portrayals of breastfeeding examined in this study are quite instructive for the viewer: while providing life force (breast milk) for your infant is empowering and a mark of ideal parenting, it's also difficult and disruptive in the current environment because of structural and cultural barriers. Efforts to improve breastfeeding rates and reduce disparities in breastfeeding and infant health require a multi-pronged strategy from many stakeholders, including the media.

Media Reactions to Breastfeeding: Reactions to Recent Headlines

Jennifer Lucas

This analysis is a comparative case study of media coverage of two recent events concerning non-private breastfeeding: a *Time* magazine cover story with a photo of a mother and breastfeeding child, and a story about an American University professor who breastfed a sick child in class. Seen in a positive light, the fact that these received coverage suggests that breastfeeding is gaining greater awareness in the U.S., which could potentially increase breastfeeding rates. Also, much of the coverage in these stories was not just about the choice to breastfeed, which was typically supported as a "non-issue." Instead, they focused on what were perceived to be "extreme" cases: attachment parenting advocates breastfeeding toddlers and a female professor breastfeeding while in class (rather than during "break" time).

Hausman (2012) notes three ways feminists might pursue critiques of breastfeeding that move beyond the medical evidence: raising awareness of social constraints, addressing structural obstacles to women's right to breastfeed, and moving beyond an ideology of a "good mother" frame. This analysis examines mediated reactions to these two stories along those thematic lines. First, media coverage is fraught with particular social expectations about women's bodies. Typically, these manifested in media presentations of these stories as "provocative" or "controversial," focusing on the most dramatic and conflictual elements of the stories. The stories tended to catalog the "visceral" reactions to these by various sources, particularly a narrative of sexual deviance related to exposed breasts and toddlers suckling on the cover of *Time* magazine. Despite many students reacted positively in the AU case, much of the media coverage focused on a student's negative tweet about the incident, and the conflict between the professor and the student newspaper.

Second, media coverage of these incidents ignored structural obstacles to realizing women's right to breastfeed. The AU example reveals important holes in support for parents, even among relatively privileged women. At the same time, much of the commentary focused on why the professor did not realize that she was being "unprofessional" by breastfeeding while she was doing her job. This raises a potentially interesting question for feminists about the borders between private and professional, and the extent to which work/family policy should orient towards balancing the two versus reconciling them.

Few media commentaries addressed the extent to which attachment parenting might be linked to social and economic privilege. Lastly, media reactions to these stories tended to reinforce the problematic theme of judging who are "good mothers," remaining focused on the specifics of the situation and the individual choices of the mothers, while implicitly suggesting each are broadly controversial. This furthers the idea of the "Mommy Wars" furthering divisiveness among mothers. Much of the discussions centered around judging whether both the AU professor and the mother on the cover of time were giving sufficient thought to common sense options for childcare and the psychological health of their children, respectively.

Negative stereotypes within the discussion were clear that feminists and "lactivists" were part of the problem, encouraging extremist views of breastfeeding and allegedly promoting them at the expense of children and fairness.

Even the AU professor sought to separate herself from "lactivists" in her own blog posting. Overall, an examination of the media reactions to these stories reveals that the media tends to highlight the extremes of the debate, obscuring the real difficulties of mothers, and furthering narratives of public breastfeeding as "provocative" rather than the norm.

By simultaneously focusing on extreme of the debate and the specifics the particular subject of the article, the media obscures contextual factors, particularly the structural lack of support for new mothers in the U.S. The analysis also suggests that negative stereotypes about activists can be seen subtly throughout the media coverage, which might influence framing by activists. In conclusion, the media's support for employing the "good mother" frame, while ignoring the social and structural constraints on women's exercise of their rights in pursuit of reproductive justice, suggests that framing of breastfeeding in the media is still more bad news than good.

Defeating the Formula Death Star, One Tweet at a Time: Using Social Media to Advocate for the WHO Code

Jeanette McCulloch and Amber McCann

Reaching breastfeeding women today means being savvy about the use of social media. While breastfeeding organizations, long without sufficient marketing resources, are recognizing the importance and increasing online efforts, formula companies are better-funded and are doing an incredibly effective job of reaching mothers using the Internet. Nestlé, in particular, has launched a well-funded social media training center that puts all its efforts into impacting the public perception of Nestlé—and undermining women's breastfeeding efforts. This "Formula Death Star," though, is not going unchallenged. Using the capacity of social media for advocates to educate and mobilize concerned consumers, a rag-tag group of rebel forces—online WHO Code activists—are working to protect the WHO Code and breastfeeding mothers everywhere.

Meeting Women Where They Are Means Using Social Media

Social media represents a revolution in communications that rivals the introduction of the printing press. Ninety-three percent of the "Millennial Generation" (those born after 1982, who have come of age in a time of dependence upon technology) are communicating online (Howe, 2000), and in the United States, for example, nearly three out of four Millennials are using a social networking website, such as Facebook, Twitter, or Pinterest (Lenhart, Purchell, Smith, & Zickuhr, 2010). Social media is widely accessed by women, ages 18 to 29, regardless of race, ethnicity, or socioeconomic status.

These changes are having a significant impact on how we talk about, learn about, and share information around birth and breastfeeding. More than half of all women responding to one survey expressed their intention to share their labor and birth experience, as it happens, on social media (Stevens, 2011). Moreover, time online increases after the birth; 44% of U.S. women spend more time online after a new baby is born, and the likelihood that a new mother will seek breastfeeding information and support online is high (Bartholomew, Schoppe-Sullivan, Glassman, Kamp Dush, & Sullivan, 2012).

Women are Seeking Information about Health Care—Including Breastfeeding—Online

Research tell us that health care providers continue to be the first choice for most people with health concerns, but online resources, including advice from peers, are a significant source of health information in the United States (Fox & Jones, 2009). Eighty percent of U.S. Internet users have sought health care information online (Fox & Jones, 2009), and birth and related topics are an area of focus. Consumers using social media are not only seeking information online, but are sharing their knowledge with others. As connectivity soars through increased Internet access and the rise of the smartphone (Smith, 2012), so does altruistic sharing of what mothers learn online (Kvedar & Kibbe, 2009).

Formula marketers are fully aware of these changes. As advocates for breastfeeding mothers, we argue that it is our responsibility to understand these changes. We also can take advantage of the unparalleled opportunities that social media provides for advocacy organizations to engage in dialogues with mothers and affect change.

What is the WHO Code?

The International Code of Marketing of Breast-milk Substitutes (World Health Organization, 1981), commonly called the "WHO Code," was written with the goal of reducing the impact of predatory marketing worldwide of formula and related products to new and expectant mothers.

The Code was written and adopted in 1981 by the World Health Organization by a vote of 118 to one (United States was the lone dissenting vote). Thirty-two countries have adopted the Code as national law, with 76 others adopting portions of the Code. Ethically and morally, the Code should be considered worldwide, even where it has not yet been adopted as law (Escobar, 2013).

Despite common misconceptions, the Code does not limit access to the use of formula or related products. The Code addresses marketing, and for good reason. When marketing spending on formula goes up, breastfeeding rates go down (Forbes, 2011).

Formula Companies Are Making Significant Investments in Social Media

Savvy institutions understand what we'd teach you in any Social Media 101 presentation: social media is an unprecedented tool for listening to and engaging with an audience. Nestlé has become a leading example of the use of social media both to reach consumers and to manage conflict and dissent.

Nestlé is the world's largest food company and also one of the world's most controversial (Mettera, 2013). Nestlé was founded on the formulation of artificial infant milk, made of cow's milk, wheat flour, and sugar (Nestlé Corporation, n.d.).

But they are not alone in their use of social media to reach parents. Research conducted in 2011, before Nestlé doubled their social media budget, found that 10 out of 11 infant formula brands commonly available in the U.S. have a social media presence. Examples of their use included Facebook pages, Twitter accounts, YouTube channels, mobile apps, sponsored reviews on blogs, and interactive web sites (Abrahams, 2012).

How Do the TOP Breastfeeding Profiles Stack Up?

Nestlé and other formula companies have built these audiences using significant budgets. While overall marketing budgets are not generally available, at least $50 million was spent on formula advertising in 2004 (Forbes, 2011), and Nestlé has been quoted as saying that they have doubled their social media spending in recent years (Thomasson, 2012). Compare this to the resources of top breastfeeding organizations, groups like La Leche League International, which is by far the best-resourced breastfeeding organization in the U.S. In 2011, LLL International had total revenues of $1.5 million and spent a little over $115,000 on "public relations, external relations, and advocacy" (La Leche League International, n.d.).

Other organizations, like KellyMom, Best for Babes Foundation, and the relatively new Breastfeeding USA have small budgets and rely largely on volunteer efforts. The result? Although, each of these organizations makes a significant impact on the women they reach, the combined number of Facebook followers for these three organizations–about 110,000 total, as of this writing–pales in comparison to that of Nestlé Good Start at five million followers (Gerber, n.d.).

Rebel Forces vs. The Death Star

Nestlé has combined its significant financial resources with social media experts and tools that have made it a shining example of how corporations should handle social media. Nestlé's "Digital Acceleration Team" has a trained staff monitoring each and every mention of Nestlé's brands. Team members identify negative "emerging issues" based on the volume of mentions and respond to those with a high level of engagement using a scripted playbook for team members (NestleCorporate, 2012).

The Formula Death Star, as it has become known to WHO Code activists, can feel overwhelming, both because it limits our capacity to reach families and because it can feel impossible to influence change at the world's largest food company.

Expanding and Improving Media Support for Breastfeeding

However, Nestlé developed these tools in response to their inability to manage an onslaught of angry advocates and consumers on social media. In 2010, Greenpeace activists were able to secure significant changes in how Nestlé sources palm oil, all thanks to a YouTube video spoof that garnered over 1.5 million views, along with a resulting social media campaign that netted more than 200,000 email complaints (Van Grove, 2010). Policy change at Nestlé based on calls from consumers is possible.

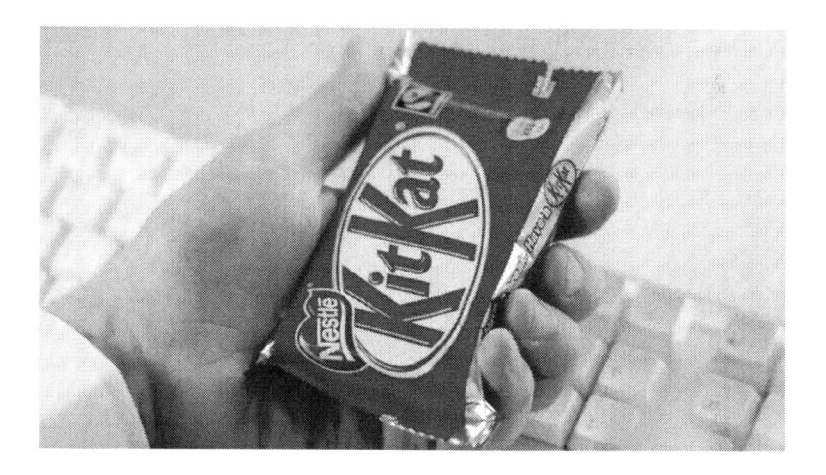

https://www.youtube.com/watch?v=1BCA8dQfGi0

Examples of Efforts to Support the WHO Code Online

Although Nestlé may have the Death Star, rebel forces are pulling together to provide much needed social media support for the WHO Code.

A recent campaign demonstrates the power of using social media tools to organize individuals, even without an official organizing body like Greenpeace. A blog post (Babendure, 2012) sparked outrage among activists when it exposed the Pan American Health Office (PAHO), the regional representative in the Americas for the World Health Organization, for accepting more than $150,000 in donations from Nestlé; the fox was helping to buy the hen house. Within days, a private Facebook group experienced rapid growth to 400 members, now at 900 members as of this writing (Friends of the WHO Code, n.d.). Each day, members were given specific action steps, including suggested scripts for tweets directed at PAHO and WHO (McCann, 2012). Members provided impromptu trainings on Twitter use and etiquette, researched the money trail, and quickly developed a strategy, including a decision to target WHO and call for a rejection of the Nestlé funding.

The result: a relatively small group of consumers and advocates, through the use of Facebook and Twitter alone, were able to force the World Health Organization to respond. But more importantly, advocates began to organize and mobilize a group of motivated individuals who will come to the next battle even more organized and prepared to engage.

How the Rebel Forces Can Defeat the Death Star

As these examples show, social media provides advocates with a unique opportunity to influence how companies do business. With ongoing support to the rebel forces, much-needed pressure can be applied to Nestlé to change their policies. But this will not come without significant work. Some areas that need support:

- Ongoing Consumer Support and Education around the WHO Code

In our anecdotal experience, mothers generally are unaware of the WHO Code, or if they are aware, they think that it limits access to formula (rather than limiting marketing of breast-milk substitutes). The importance of the WHO Code needs to be distilled into social-media-friendly images and infographics to build awareness and support for future efforts.

- Ongoing Education of Maternal Health Advocates

The WHO Code impacts more than just breastfeeding. Anyone concerned with infant and maternal health should be aware of and providing support for the adoptions and enforcement of the WHO Code worldwide.

- Bring Even More Social Media Savvy to the Table

After Nestlé's run-in with Greenpeace, they hired a top-notch social media strategist to revamp their approach and train the digital engagement team. Nestlé uses sophisticated tools to monitor and respond to issues. The Friends of the WHO Code—and any group hoping to use social media for im-

It Takes a Village

pact—needs people on hand who are savvy in the use of social media and the funding for at least some basic tools to help make the job collaborative.

- Keep Doing What We Know Best

One the greatest impacts of the PAHO/WHO crisis was to bring together the community that will need to continue to take action. This and other groups need to use traditional community organizing strategies along with social media as the tools they use to create a more level playing field.

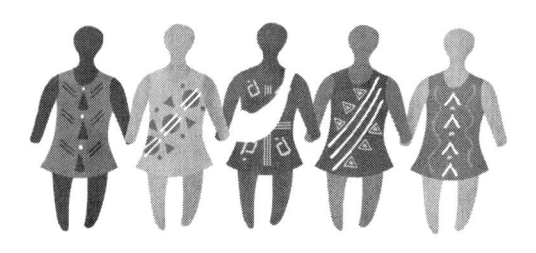

Contributors*

Sheryl Abrahams, MPH, is currently a DrPH student in the Division of Health Promotion and Behavioral Science at the University of Texas School of Public Health. She works as a Research and Development Associate with the Carolina Global Breastfeeding Institute, Global School of Public Health, UNC Chapel Hill, Chapel Hill, North Carolina.

Erica Hesch Anstey, MA, CLC, is pursuing her doctorate in Public Health at the University of South Florida in Tampa, Florida

Emily Anzicek, PhD, is an instructor and the Director of the Introduction to Communication course in the Department of Communication at Bowling Green State University in Ohio.

Shobha Arole, PhD, is Director of the Comprehensive Rural Health Project in Jamkhed, India. She is also an ordained minister and honorary presbyter in the Jamkhed Community Church.

Helen Ball, PhD, is Professor of Anthropology at Durham University, England, where she runs the Parent-Infant Sleep Lab.

Margaret Bentley, PhD, is the Carla Smith Chamblee Distinguished Professor in the Department of Nutrition, Associate Dean for Global Health, and the Associate Director, Institute for Global Health and Infectious Disease, in the Gillings Global School of Public Health, University of North Carolina at Chapel Hill, Chapel Hill, North Carolina.

Anna Blair, PhD, IBCLC, CLC, is the Director of Academic Programs at the Healthy Children Project, East Sandwich, Massachusetts. She is also chair of the Department of Maternal and Child Health, Lactation Consulting at Union Institute and University, a "university without walls" headquartered in Cincinnati, Ohio.

Lindsey Bickers Bock, MPH, is the program manager for the Working Well project at NC Prevention Partners, Chapel Hill, North Carolina.

Jessye Brick is a Master's in Public Health Candidate in the Maternal and Child Health Department in the Gillings Global School of Public Health, at the University of North Carolina at Chapel Hill. She is currently working to identify emerging opportunities for local health departments at the North Carolina Institute for Public Health, Chapel Hill, North Carolina.

Kajsa Brimdyr, PhD, is an affiliated faculty member and advisor for the Maternal Child Health: Lactation Consulting bachelor's degree at Union Institute and University. Dr. Brimdyr is the Director of Operations for Healthy Children, a non-profit 501(c)3 on Cape Cod, MA, where she is also on the faculty and a researcher.

Cynthia Bulik, PhD, FAED, is Distinguished Professor of Eating Disorders, Professor of Nutrition, and Associate Director, Center of Genomics, Gillings School of Global Public Health, University of North Carolina at Chapel Hill, Chapel Hill, North Carolina.

Natalie Smith Carlson, MA, is a lecturer at North Dakota State University in both the English and Women's and Gender Studies Departments, where she teaches courses like Writing in the Health Professions and Introduction to Women's Studies.

Amanda Barnes Cook is a PhD candidate in Political Science and Political Theory at the University of North Carolina at Chapel Hill, Chapel Hill, North Carolina.

Debra Brandon, PhD, RN, CCNS, FAAN, is Associate Professor of Nursing, School of Nursing, Duke University, Durham, NC.

It Takes a Village

Karin Cadwell, PhD, FAAN, RN, IBCLC, is the Executive Director and Lead Faculty of Healthy Children.

Ginny Combs, MSN, RNC-MNN, IBCLC, is the Mother-Baby Unit Manager, Boston Medical Center and with the Lactation and Baby Café at Codman Square Health Center, Boston, Massachusetts.

Carole Dobrich, IBCLC, is the Senior Lactation Consultant and educator at the HFPC-Goldfarb Breastfeeding Clinic in Montreal, a tertiary-level lactation center. She is co-owner of The International Institute of Human Lactation Inc., with her colleague Dr. Lenore Goldfarb. Carole also volunteers for INFACT Quebec, a non-profit organization that aims to protect and normalize breastfeeding in Quebec.

Sally Dowling, MS, PhD, became a Member of the Faculty of Public Health of the Royal College of Physicians, London in 2006. She works as a Senior Lecturer at the University of the West of England, Bristol, UK.

Emily Dunn, CLC, DONA, is a graduate student and research associate in the Departments of Community & Family Health and Anthropology at the University of South Florida. She is pursuing a dual master's degree with concentrations in maternal and child health and biocultural medical anthropology. She is also vice president of the USF Maternal and Child Health Student Organization and a member of the Hillsborough County Breastfeeding Taskforce.

Contributors

Eugenia (Geni) Eng, DrPH, MPH, is Professor of Health Behavior and Health Education and Director of the Kellogg Health Scholars Postdoctoral Program at the University of North Carolina at Chapel Hill, Gillings School of Global Public Health, Chapel Hill, North Carolina.

Camille Fabiyi, MPH, is currently a PhD candidate in the Maternal & Child Health program at University of Illinois at Chicago (UIC). Ms. Fabiyi also serves as project director at the UIC College of Nursing on a NIH funded multi-site study examining the impact of a developmental intervention on mother-premature infant dyads at social risk.

Katherine Foss, PhD, is an Assistant Professor at Middle Tennessee State University, where she teaches courses in women and the media, health communication, and entertainment studies.

Bette Gebrian, BS, PhD, MPH, is a public health nurse and medical anthropologist who has lived and worked in rural Haiti for the past 25 years.

Connie Gates, MPH, works with Comprehensive Rural Health Project (CRHP), Jamkhed, India. In India and in the U.S., she is representative of CRHP and director of Jamkhed International-North America.

Barbara Goldman, PhD, is Senior Scientist and Director, Behavioral Measurement Core and Audio-Visual Resource Center, Frank Porter Graham Child Development Institute,

University of North Carolina at Chapel Hill, Chapel Hill, North Carolina.

Reyna Gordon, PhD, is a Research Fellow at the Vanderbilt Kennedy Center, where she uses psychophysiological methods, such as electroencephalography, to study language and music cognition in individuals with disabilities and typical development.

Jane Grassley, PhD, IBCLC, joined the Boise State University School of Nursing faculty in 2010. She also holds a joint appointment with Women's Services at St. Luke's Regional Health System to collaboratively develop research projects with the Treasure Valley hospitals' lactation consultants.

Talene Ghazarian is a Master in Public Health Candidate in the Maternal and Child Health Department, Gillings Global School of Public Health at the University of North Carolina at Chapel Hill. Currently, she is working at the North Carolina Institute for Public Health (NCHIP), where she is helping to identify contextual changes and potential opportunities for local health departments in North Carolina.

Tyra Toston Gross is a doctoral candidate at the University of Georgia, College of Public Health. Tyra is also completing graduate certificates in Global Health, Nonprofit Management, and Qualitative Research at UGA, Athens, Georgia.

Emily Healy, IBCLC, is a lactation consultant at Seattle Breastfeeding Medicine and a member of the Puget Sound Perinatal Collaborative, a group of organizations working to counter institutional racism in perinatal support to better meet the needs of families of color in Washington State. She was the co-coordinator of the "Inequity in Breastfeeding Support Summit; The Impact of Institutional Racism, Power, and White Privilege on Breastfeeding Rates and Maternal Infant Health" (Held in Seattle June of 2013).

Alison Higgins is the training volunteer with the Comprehensive Rural Health Project in Jamkhed, India.

Eric Hodges, PhD, FNP-BC, is Associate Professor and Interim Director of Behavior Laboratory, School of Nursing, at the University of North Carolina at Chapel Hill, Chapel Hill, North Carolina.

Diane Holditch-Davis, PhD, RN, FAAN, is the Marcus E. Hobbs Distinguished Professor of Nursing, School of Nursing, Duke University, Durham, North Carolina.

Tamisha F. Johnson, MD, is Maternal Health Projects Coordinator at the Bureau of Maternal, Infant and Reproductive Health in the New York City Department of Health and Mental Hygiene. She is currently completing her Master's Degree in Public Health at CUNY Hunter College.

Ghada Khan is a doctor of public health candidate at the George Washington University, School of Public Health and Health Services in Fairfax, Virginia.

Panagiota Kitsantas, PhD, is Associate Professor of Biostatistics and Epidemiology in Health Administration and Policy, College of Health and Human Services, George Mason University, Fairfax, Virginia.

Miriam H. Labbok, MD, MPH, IBCLC, FACPM, FABM, FILCA, is Professor and Director of Carolina Global Breastfeeding Institute Department of Maternal and Child Health, Gillings School of Global Public Health, University of North Carolina at Chapel Hill, Chapel Hill, North Carolina. She is co-director of the Breastfeeding and Feminism International Conference. Along with Drs. Paige Hall Smith and Bernice Hausman, she edited the 2012 book, *Beyond Health, Beyond Choice: Breastfeeding Constraints and Realities*, which was based on presentations at the 2010 Breastfeeding and Feminism Symposium.

Taylor Livingston is a PhD candidate in the Department of Anthropology at the University of North Carolina at Chapel Hill, Chapel Hill, North Carolina.

Judy Lewis, MPhil, is Professor Emeritus of the University of Connecticut Health Center and with Global Health Consulting in Hartford, Connecticut.

Jennifer Lucas, PhD, is Associate Professor of Politics at Saint Anselm College, where she teaches courses in American government, women and politics, congressional politics, and peace and social justice.

Cynthia Good Mojab, MS, LMHCA, IBCLC, RLC, CATSM, is Director of Life Circle Counseling and Consulting, LLC.

Contributors

Amy Meador, MPH, joined NC Prevention Partners in 2011. She is the program manager for the Wellness Research Council, which leverages data from NC Prevention Partners' proprietary online assessment, WorkHealthy AmericaSM, and partnerships with research experts to answer the question of what works best in worksite wellness.

Amber McCann, IBCLC, is co-editor of Lactation Matters, the International Lactation Consultant Association's official blog. She has written for a number of other breastfeeding support blogs, including for Hygeia, The Leaky Boob, and Best for Babes, and is a regular contributor to The Boob Group, a weekly online radio program for breastfeeding mothers.

Deborah McCarter-Spaulding, PhD, RN, IBCLC, WHNP-BC, is an Associate Professor at Saint Anselm College in Manchester, NH, where she teaches childbearing in both the classroom and the clinical setting.

Jeanette McCulloch, IBCLC, is a co-founder of BirthSwell, a community of birth and breastfeeding professionals using social media and communication skills to spread evidence-based information to women. After helping to launch the freeourmidwives.com campaign in New York, she recently joined the Citizens for Midwifery board as the communications chair.

Vi Nguyen, MS, is with the Department of Health Administration and Policy, College of Health and Human Services, George Mason University, Fairfax, Virginia.

Kathy Parry, MPH, IBCLC, joined the Carolina Global Breastfeeding Institute, in the Department of Maternal and Child Health, Gillings School of Global Public Health, University of North Carolina at Chapel Hill, Chapel Hill, North Carolina in May of 2012 after two years as graduate research assistant with the Institute.

Aunchalee Palmquist, PhD, is Assistant Professor of Anthropology at Elon University, Elon, North Carolina.

Yosef Pandit, DCHD, is Mobile Operations Manager with the Comprehensive Rural Health Project in Jamkhed, India.

Eliana Perrin, MD, is Associate Professor, Division of General Pediatrics and Adolescent Medicine, Department of Pediatrics, School of Medicine, University of North Carolina at Chapel Hill.

Martin P. Ward Platt, MB, ChB, MD, FRCP, FRCPCH, is consulting pediatrician working at the Royal Victoria Infirmary at Newcastle upon Tyne, Honorary Clinical Reader in neonatal and paediatric medicine at Newcastle University, and Clinical Director of the northern Regional Maternity Survey Office.

Debra Prosnitz, MPH, is Associate Technical Specialist with ICF International.

Jennifer Proto is a senior undergraduate studying public health studies and anthropology at Elon University, Elon North Carolina.

Contributors

Mika Putterman is the Founder of Montreal Milk Share in Montreal, Canada

Sarah Davis Redman, MA, has a master's degree in public affairs from the University of Texas at Austin, and is currently a PhD candidate at the University of Illinois at Chicago.

Paige Hall Smith, MSPH, PhD, is Associate Professor of Public Health Education and Director the Center for Women's Health and Wellness at the University of North Carolina at Greensboro, USA. She is founder and co-director of the Breastfeeding and Feminism International Conference. Along with Drs. Bernice Hausman and Miriam Labbok, she edited the 2012 book, *Beyond Health, Beyond Choice: Breastfeeding Constraints and Realities*, which was based on presentations at the 2010 Breastfeeding and Feminism Symposium.

Taylor Marie Snyder is a Master in Public Health (MPH) Candidate in the Maternal and Child Health Department at the University of North Carolina at Chapel Hill. She is currently a Graduate Research Consultant at the North Carolina Institute for Public Health (NCHIP).

Chirayath Suchindran is Professor and Director of Graduate Studies, Department of Biostatistics, Gillings School of Global Public Health, , University of North Carolina at Chapel Hill, Chapel Hill, North Carolina.

Pushpa Sutar is Director of Padali Model Villages with the Comprehensive Rural Health Project in Jamkhed, India.

Emily Taylor, MPH, CD(DONA), is the Deputy Director of, the Carolina Global Breastfeeding Institute at the University of North Carolina at Chapel Hill. Emily serves as the Secretary of the Board of the United States Breastfeeding Committee and the Chair of the North Carolina Breastfeeding Coalition.

Erin N. Taylor, PhD, is an Associate Professor of Political Science at Western Illinois University.

Amanda Thompson, PhD, is Associate Professor, Department of Anthropology, University of North Carolina at Chapel Hill, Chapel Hill, North Carolina.

Cecilia Tomori, PhD, recently earned her PhD in Anthropology, with a focus in medical anthropology, from the University of Michigan. She is presently working on applying her anthropological training in the field of HIV prevention at the Johns Hopkins Bloomberg School of Public Health, Baltimore, Maryland.

Cynthia Turner-Maffei, MA, ALC, IBCLC, is lead faculty and lactation consultant at the Healthy Children's Center for Breastfeeding, East Sandwich, Massachusetts.

Kristin Tully, PhD, studied Biological Anthropology at Durham University in the United Kingdom. She is currently a postdoctoral fellow through the Carolina Consortium on Human Development at the Center for Developmental Science through University of North Carolina at Chapel Hill and Duke University, Durham, North Carolina.

Contributors

Kirsten Unfried is an analyst with ICF International whose responsibilities include supporting analyses of data drawn from the client's portfolio of grants, maintaining a project database, and supporting grantees in their use of small-sample population-based surveys.

Lora Ebert Wallace, PhD, is Associate Professor of Sociology at Western Illinois University.

Heather Wasser, RN, CLC, is a doctoral student and the project director of a multi-component obesity prevention intervention targeting African American families in central North Carolina, Mothers and Others: Family-Based Obesity Prevention for Infants and Toddlers. This project is housed in the Gillings Global School of Public Health, University of North Carolina at Chapel Hill, Chapel Hill, North Carolina.

Beryl Watnick, PhD, is the Dean of the Bachelor of Science Programs at Union Institute & University. Beryl came to the university in 2001 to develop the Master of Education, which was designed to fulfill the requirements for educator certification.

Jacqueline H. Wolf, PhD, is Professor of the History of Medicine and chair of the Department of Social Medicine at Ohio University.

Jennifer Yourkavitch, MPH, CLC, is Senior Technical Specialist with ICF International.

It Takes a Village

Erin A. Wagner, MS, served as a Peace Corps volunteer in the Dominican Republic until 2010, working to promote community health, particularly in the areas of food security, reproductive health, and maternal and infant nutrition. She now works at Cincinnati Children's Hospital Center for Interdisciplinary Research in Human Milk and Lactation as a research coordinator.

*Affiliations presented areas per submission at the 2013 conference

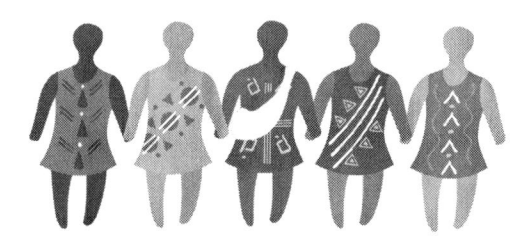

References

Introduction

Labbok, M., Smith, P.H., & Taylor, E. (2008). Breastfeeding and feminism: A focus on reproductive health, rights and justice. *International Breastfeeding Journal, 3:8*, doi:10.1186/1746-4358-3-8

Smith, P.H., Hausman, B.L., & Labbok, M. (2012). *Beyond health, beyond choice: Breastfeeding constraints and realities.* New Brunswick, NJ: Rutgers University Press.

Chapter 1

It Takes a Village: Latest Thinking on Community-Based Participatory Approaches to Behavior Change

Bandura, A. (1997). *Self-efficacy: The exercise of control.* New York: W.H. Freeman and Company.

Bramson, L., Lee, J. W., Moore, E., Montgomery, S., Neish, C., & Bahjri, K. (2010). Effect of early skin-to-skin contact during the first 3 hours following birth on exclusive breastfeeding during the maternity hospital stay. *Journal of Human Lactation, 26*(2), 130-137. doi: 10.1177/08903344093555779

Creedy, D. K., Dennis, C., Blyth, R., Moyle, W., Pratt, J., & De Vries, S. M. (2003). Psychometric characteristics of the Breastfeeding Self-Efficacy Scale: Data from an Australian sample. *Research in Nursing and Health, 26*(2), 143-152.

Dennis, C. (2003). The Breastfeeding Self-Efficacy Scale: Psychometric assessment of the short form. *JOGNN: Journal of Obstetric, Gynecologic and Neonatal Nursing, 32*(6), 734-744.

Field, T. (2010). Postpartum depression effects on early interactions, parenting, and safety practices: A review. *Infant Behavior and Development, 33*(1), 1-6.

Grassley, J., & Eschiti, V. (2008). Grandmother breastfeeding support: What do mothers need and want? *Birth: Issues in Perinatal Care, 35*(4), 329-335.

References

Gregory, A., Penrose, K., Morrison, C., Dennis, C., & MacArthur, C. (2008). Psychometric properties of the Breastfeeding Self-Efficacy Scale-Short Form in an ethnically diverse U.K. sample. *Public Health Nursing, 25*(3), 278-284.

Hannula, L., Kaunonen, M., & Tarkka, M. (2008). A systematic review of professional support interventions for breastfeeding. *Journal of Clinical Nursing, 17*(9), 1132-1143. doi: http://dx.doi.org/10.1111/j.1365-2702.2007.02239.x

Kaunonen, M., Hannula, L., & Tarkka, M.T. (2012). A systematic review of peer support interventions for breastfeeding. *Journal of Clinical Nursing, 21*(13/14), 1943-1954. doi: http://dx.doi.org/10.1111/j.1365-2702.2012.04071.x

McCarter-Spaulding, D., & Gore, R. (2009). Breastfeeding self-efficacy in women of African descent. *JOGNN: Journal of Obstetric, Gynecologic & Neonatal Nursing, 38*(2), 230-243.

McCarter-Spaulding, D., & Gore, R. (2012). Social support improves breastfeeding self-efficacy in a sample of Black women. *Clinical Lactation, 3*(3), 114-117.

Mossman, M., Heaman, M., Dennis, C.-L., & Morris, M. (2008). The influence of adolescent mothers' breastfeeding confidence and attitudes on breastfeeding initiation and duration. *Journal of Human Lactation, 24*(3), 268-277. doi: 10.1177/0890334408316075

Phillips, K. E. (2011). First-time breastfeeding mothers: Perceptions and lived experiences with breastfeeding. *International Journal of Childbirth Education, 26*(3), 1720.

Strong, G. D. (2011). Provider management and support for breastfeeding pain. *Journal of Obstetric, Gynecologic, and Neonatal Nursing, 40*, 753-764. doi: 10.1111/j.1552-6909.2011.01303.x

Torres, M. M., Torres, R. R. D., Rodriguez, A. M. P., & Dennis, C. (2003). Translation and validation of the Breastfeeding Self-Efficacy Scale into Spanish: Data from a Puerto Rican population. *Journal of Human Lactation, 19*(1), 35-42.

Wolfberg, A. J., Michels, K. B., Shields, W., O'Campo, P., Bronner, Y., & Bienstock, J. (2004). Dads as breastfeeding advocates: Results from a randomized controlled trial of an educational intervention. *American Journal of Obstetrics and Gynecology, 191*(3), 708-712.

Wutke, K., & Dennis, C. (2007). The reliability and validity of the Polish version of the Breastfeeding Self-Efficacy Scale-Short Form: Translation and psychometric assessment. *International Journal of Nursing Studies, 44*(8), 1439-1446.

Does it Really Take a Village? Self-efficacy and Social Support Theory and Research

References

Bandura, A. (1997). *Self-efficacy: The exercise of control.* New York: W.H. Freeman and Company.

Bramson, L., Lee, J. W., Moore, E., Montgomery, S., Neish, C., & Bahjri, K. (2010). Effect of early skin-to-skin contact during the first 3 hours following birth on exclusive breastfeeding during the maternity hospital stay. *Journal of Human Lactation, 26*(2), 130-137. doi: 10.1177/08903344093555779

Creedy, D. K., Dennis, C., Blyth, R., Moyle, W., Pratt, J., & De Vries, S. M. (2003). Psychometric characteristics of the Breastfeeding Self-Efficacy Scale: Data from an Australian sample. *Research in Nursing and Health, 26*(2), 143-152.

Dennis, C. (2003). The Breastfeeding Self-Efficacy Scale: Psychometric assessment of the short form. *JOGNN: Journal of Obstetric, Gynecologic and Neonatal Nursing, 32*(6), 734-744.

Field, T. (2010). Postpartum depression effects on early interactions, parenting, and safety practices: A review. *Infant Behavior and Development, 33*(1), 1-6.

Grassley, J., & Eschiti, V. (2008). Grandmother breastfeeding support: What do mothers need and want? *Birth: Issues in Perinatal Care, 35*(4), 329-335.

Gregory, A., Penrose, K., Morrison, C., Dennis, C., & MacArthur, C. (2008). Psychometric properties of the Breastfeeding Self-Efficacy Scale-Short Form in an ethnically diverse U.K. sample. *Public Health Nursing, 25*(3), 278-284.

Hannula, L., Kaunonen, M., & Tarkka, M. (2008). A systematic review of professional support interventions for breastfeeding. *Journal of Clinical Nursing, 17*(9), 1132-1143. doi: http://dx.doi.org/10.1111/j.1365-2702.2007.02239.x

Kaunonen, M., Hannula, L., & Tarkka, M.T. (2012). A systematic review of peer support interventions for breastfeeding. *Journal of Clinical Nursing, 21*(13/14), 1943-1954. doi: http://dx.doi.org/10.1111/j.1365-2702.2012.04071.x

McCarter-Spaulding, D., & Gore, R. (2009). Breastfeeding self-efficacy in women of African descent. *JOGNN: Journal of Obstetric, Gynecologic & Neonatal Nursing, 38*(2), 230-243.

McCarter-Spaulding, D., & Gore, R. (2012). Social support improves breastfeeding self-efficacy in a sample of Black women. *Clinical Lactation, 3*(3), 114-117.

Mossman, M., Heaman, M., Dennis, C.-L., & Morris, M. (2008). The influence of adolescent mothers' breastfeeding confidence and attitudes on breastfeeding initiation and duration. *Journal of Human Lactation, 24*(3), 268-277. doi: 10.1177/0890334408316075

References

Phillips, K. E. (2011). First-time breastfeeding mothers: Perceptions and lived experiences with breastfeeding. *International Journal of Childbirth Education, 26*(3), 1720.

Strong, G. D. (2011). Provider management and support for breastfeeding pain. *Journal of Obstetric, Gynecologic, and Neonatal Nursing, 40*, 753-764. doi: 10.1111/j.1552-6909.2011.01303.x

Torres, M. M., Torres, R. R. D., Rodriguez, A. M. P., & Dennis, C. (2003). Translation and validation of the Breastfeeding Self-Efficacy Scale into Spanish: Data from a Puerto Rican population. *Journal of Human Lactation, 19*(1), 35-42.

Wolfberg, A. J., Michels, K. B., Shields, W., O'Campo, P., Bronner, Y., & Bienstock, J. (2004). Dads as breastfeeding advocates: Results from a randomized controlled trial of an educational intervention. *American Journal of Obstetrics and Gynecology, 191*(3), 708-712.

Wutke, K., & Dennis, C. (2007). The reliability and validity of the Polish version of the Breastfeeding Self-Efficacy Scale-Short Form: Translation and psychometric assessment. *International Journal of Nursing Studies, 44*(8), 1439-1446.

It Takes a Village

Breastfeeding and the Status of Women

Centers for Disease Control and Prevention. (2013). *Breastfeeding report card 2013*. Retrieved from: http://www.cdc.gov/breastfeeding/data/reportcard.htm#Outcome.

IBM Corp. (2012). *IBM SPSS Statistics for Windows, Version 21.0*. Armonk, NY: IBM Corp.

Smith, P. H. (2012). Breastfeeding promotion through gender equity. In P. H. Smith, B.L. Hausman, and M. Labbok (Eds.), *Breastfeeding constraints and realities* (pp. 25-35). New Brunswick, NJ: Rutgers University Press.

Van Esterik, P. (1989). *Beyond the breast-bottle controversy.* New Brunswick, NJ: Rutgers University Press.

The Inadequate Breast: Medical and Social Origins of Breastfeeding Myths

Abt, I. A. (1904, April 24). Domestic science conducted by the School of Domestic Arts and Science of Chicago Lesson No. 212—Milk Commission. *Chicago Tribune, 16*.

Are Infant Feeding Methods Changing. (1931). *Public Health Nursing, 23*, 581-85.

References

Brennemann, J. (1938). Periods in the life of the American Pediatric Society: Adolescence, 1900-1915. *Transactions of the American Pediatrics Society, 50*, 56-67. Bulletin Chicago School of Sanitary Instruction (June 3, 1911).

Clarke, E. H. (1873). *Sex in education; or a fair chance for girls.* Boston: James R. Osgood & Co.

FEMA (2004). *Food and water in an emergency. American Red Cross*, U.S. Department of Agriculture. Retrieved from: http://www.fema.gov/pdf/library/f&web.pdf.

Levenstein, H. (1983). "Best for babies" or "preventable infanticide"? The controversy over artificial feeding of infants in America, 1880-1920. *Journal of American History, 70*, 75-94.

Mother's Parliament. (1886). *Babyhood,* 175-76.

Rotch, T. M. (1890). The management of human breast-milk in cases of difficult infantile digestion. *Transactions of the American Pediatric Society, 2*, 88-100.

Rotch, T. M. (1896). *Pediatrics: The hygienic and medical treatment of children.* Philadelphia: J. B. Lippincott Company.

Rotch, T. M. (1901). The cardinal principles for the successful feeding of infants. *Interstate Medical Journal, 17*, 305-15.

Rotch, T. M. (1904). Some considerations regarding substitute feeding during the first year. *Transactions of the American Pediatrics Society, 16,* 41-55.

Salmon, M. (1994). The cultural significance of breastfeeding and infant care in early modern England and America. *Journal of Social History, 28,* 247-269.

The Youngest Member of the Family. (1889). *Arthur's Home Magazine, 59,* 107.

Tow, A. (1934). The rationale of breast feeding: A modern concept. *Hygeia, 12,* 407.

Wolf, J. H. (2000). The social and medical construction of lactation pathology. *Women and Health, 30,* 93-110.

Wolf, J. H. (2001). *Don't kill your baby: Public health and the decline of breastfeeding in the 19th and 20th Century.* Columbus: Ohio State University Press.

Wood-Allen, M. (1896). Physical nurture. *New Crusade, October,* 180-181.

Chapter 2

The Welfare State and the Breastfeeding Worker

Duberstein Lindberg, L. (1996). Women's decisions about breastfeeding and maternal employment. *Journal of Marriage and Family, 58*(1), 239-251.

References

Ellingsaeter, A. L., & Ronsen, M. (1996). The dual strategy: Motherhood and the work contract in Scandinavia. *European Journal of Population, 12*(3), 239-260.

Esping-Andersen, G. (2002). *Why we need a new welfare state.* Oxford: Oxford University Press.

Helsedirektoratet. (2008). *Spedkost – 6 måneder: Landsomfattende kostholdsundersøkelse blant 6 måneder gamle barn. Spedkost 2006-2007.* Retrieved from: <http://www.helsedirektoratet.no/vp/multimedia/archive/00054/IS-1535_54649a.pdf>

Kersting, M., & Dulon, M. (2001). Assessment of breast-feeding promotion in hospitals and follow-up survey of mother-infant pairs in Germany: The SuSe study. *Public Health Nutrition, 5*(4), 547-552.

Orloff, A. S. (1993). Gender and the social rights of citizenship: The comparative analysis of gender relations and welfare states. *American Sociological Review, 58*(3), 303-28.

Sveriges Officiella Statistik. (2007). *Amning av barn födda 2005.* Retrieved from: http://www.socialstyrelsen.se/Lists/Artikelkatalog/Attachments/9321/2007-42-12_20074212.pdf

U.K. National Health Service. (2007). *Infant Feeding Survey 2005.* Retrieved from: http://www.ic.nhs.uk/pubs/ifs2005

U.S. Centers for Disease Control and Prevention. (2010). *Breastfeeding among U.S. children born 1999—2007. CDC National Immunization Survey*. Retrieved from: http://www.cdc.gov/breastfeeding/data/NIS_data/index.htm

Williams, J. (2001). *Unbending gender: Why family and work conflict and what to do about it.* Oxford: Oxford University Press.

Breastfeeding Equity: Summary of a Concept Analysis

Bartek, M., & Reinhold, A. (2010). The burden of suboptimal breastfeeding in the United States: A pediatric cost analysis. *Pediatrics, 125*(5), 1048-1056.

Braveman, P. (2006). Health disparities and health equity: Concepts and measurement. *Annual Review Public Health, 27*, 167-194.

Cattaneo, A. (2012). Academy of Breastfeeding Medicine founder's lecture 2011: Inequalities and inequities in breastfeeding: An international perspective. *Breastfeeding Medicine, 7*(1), 3-9.

CDC. (2012). *Breastfeeding report card-United States, 2012. 1-4*. Retrieved from: http://www.cdc.gov/breastfeeding/pdf/2012BreastfeedingReportCard.pdf

References

Kukla, R. (2006). Ethics and ideology in breastfeeding advocacy campaigns. *Hypatia, 21*(1), 157-180. doi: 10.2979/hyp.2006.21.1.157

Labbok, M., Smith, P. H., & Taylor, E. (2008). Breastfeeding and feminism: A focus on reproductive health, rights, and justice. *International Breastfeeding Journal, 3*(8), 1-6.

Labbok, M., & Nakaji, E. (2010). Breastfeeding: A biological, ecological, and human rights imperative for global health. In P. Murphy & C. Landford Smith (Eds.), *Women's global health and human rights* (pp. 1-556). Sudbury, MA: Jones and Bartlett.

Maxwell, R. J. (1992). Dimensions of quality revisited: From thought to action. *Quality in Health Care, 1*, 171-177.

McKinley, N. M., & Hyde, J. S. (2004). Personal attitudes or structural factors? A contextual analysis of breastfeeding duration. *Psychology of Women Quarterly, 28*(4), 388-399. doi: 10.1111/j.1471-6402.2004.00156.x

Mezirow, J., & Associates (Eds.). (1990). *Fostering critical reflection in adulthood: A guide to transformative and emancipatory learning*. San Francisco: Jossey-Bass Publishers.

Murtagh, L., & Moulton, A. (2011). Working mothers, breastfeeding, and the law. *American Journal of Public Health, 101*(2), 217-223.

U.S. DHHS. (2011). *The Surgeon General's Call to Action to Support Breastfeeding.* Washington, DC: Office of the Surgeon General. Retrieved from: http://www.surgeongeneral.gov.

Whitehead, M. (1985). *The concepts and principles of equity and health.* Copenhagen: World Health Organization. Retrieved from: http://salud.ciee.flacso.org.ar/flacso/optativas/equity_and_health.pdf.

Milk and Motherhood: Breastfeeding and "Good Motherhood" Among African American Women in the South

Anderson, J. B. (2011). *Durham County: A history of Durham County, North Carolina.* Durham, NC: Duke University Press.

Center for Disease Control and Prevention. (2011). *Breastfeeding report card-United States, 2011.* Retrieved from: http://www.cdc.gov/breastfeeding/data/reportcard.htm

Collins, P. H. (2004). *Black sexual politics: African Americans, gender, and the new racism.* New York: Routledge Press.

Fassin, D. (2007). *When bodies remember: Experiences and politics of AIDS in South Africa.* Berkeley, CA: University of California Press.

References

Hooks, B. (1987). *Talking back: Thinking feminist, thinking Black*. Cambridge: MA: South End Press.

Jordan, B. (1993). *Birth in four cultures: A cross-cultural investigation of childbirth in Yucatan, Holland, Sweden, and the United States*. Prospect Heights, IL: Waveland Press.

Labbok, M., & Taylor, E. (2010). Call to action on breastfeeding in NC: Review and rationale. *North Carolina Medical Journal, 71*(5), 459-463.

Martin, E. (1987). *The woman in the body: A cultural analysis of reproduction*. Boston: Beacon Press.

Roberts, D. (1997). *Killing the black body: Race, reproduction, and the meaning of liberty*. New York: Pantheon.

Undoing Institutional Racism in Perinatal Support Organizations: First Steps for Eliminating Racial Inequity in Breastfeeding Support

Centers for Disease Control and Prevention. (2012). *Breastfeeding report card—United States, 2012*. Atlanta, GA: Centers for Disease Control and Prevention.

Chapman, D. J., Morel, K., Anderson, A.K., Damio, G., & Perez-Escamilla, R. (2010). Breastfeeding peer counseling: From efficacy through scale-up. *Journal of Human Lactation, 26*(3), 314-326.

Collins, J. W., & David, R. J. (2009). Racial disparity in low birth weight and infant mortality. *Clinical Perinatology, 36*, 63–73.

Crossroads Anti-Racism Organizing and Training. (2007). *Crossroads anti-racism organizing and training teaching and training methodology documentation and evaluation report.* Matteson, IL: Crossroads Anti-Racism Organizing & Training.

Crossroads Anti-Racism Organizing and Training. (2011). *CALPACT Training: Introduction to institutional racism (Part One)* [Video file]. Retrieved from: http://www.youtube.com/watch?v=1xyjLwmFfJY

Good Mojab, C. (2013, June). *Unpacking the invisible diaper bag of white privilege: Deconstructing racial inequities in breastfeeding support.* Presented at the Inequity in Breastfeeding Support Summit, Seattle.

Jones, C. P. (2000). Levels of racism: A theoretic framework and a gardener's tale. *American Journal of Public Health, 90*(8), 1212–1215.

Rishel, P. E., & Sweeney, P. (2005). Comparison of breastfeeding rates among women delivering infants in military treatment facilities with and without lactation consultants. *Military Medicine, 170*(5), 435-438.

References

Seals Allers, K. (2012a). *Lactation consultants need to diversify yesterday*. August 3, 2012a. We.news. Retrieved from: http://womensenews.org

Seals Allers, K. (2012b). *Breastfeeding needs diverse advocates*. September 14, 2012b. Upi.com. Retrieved from: http://www.upi.com

Seattle Human Services Coalition. (2005). *Identifying institutional racism folio: Tools to assist human service organizations identify and eliminate institutional racism in their organization*. Seattle, WA: Seattle Human Services Coalition.

Stuebe, A. (2009). The risks of not breastfeeding for mothers and infants. *Review of Obstetrics & Gynecology, 2*(4), 222–231.

USBC. (2011). *Diversity values statement*. Retrieved from: http://www.usbreastfeeding.org

U.S. Department of Health and Human Services. (2011). *The Surgeon General's Call to Action to Support Breastfeeding*. Washington, DC: U.S. Department of Health and Human Services, Office of the Surgeon General.

Yglesia, M. (2012). *One school's journey to dismantle racism in the classroom. Association of Midwifery Educators Enews*. Retrieved from: http://associationofmidwiferyeducators.org.

Mothers and Others: An Intervention with Promise for Improving Breastfeeding Outcomes among African American Women

Bentley, M., Gavin, L., Black, M.M., & Teti, L. (1999). Infant feeding practices of low-income, African American, adolescent mothers: An ecological, multigenerational perspective. *Social Science & Medicine, 49*(8), 1085-1100. doi: S0277953699001987 [pii].

Centers for Disease Control and Prevention. (2014). *Breastfeeding report card 2014*. Retrieved from: http://www.cdc.gov/breastfeeding/pdf/2014breastfeedingreportcard.pdf

Centers for Disease Control and Prevention. (2007). *Breastfeeding among U.S. children born 2001-2011. CDC National Immunization Survey*. Retrieved from: http://www.cdc.gov/breastfeeding/data/nis_data/

De La Mora, A., & Russell, D.W. (1999). The Iowa Infant Feeding Attitude Scale: Analysis of reliability and validity. *Journal of Applied Social Psychology, 29*(11), 2362-2417.

Dennis, C.L. (2003). The breastfeeding self-efficacy scale: Psychometric assessment of the short form. *Journal of Obstetric, Gynecology, & Neonatal Nursing, 32*(6), 734-744.

References

DiGirolamo, A., Thompson, N., Martorell, R., Fein, S., & Grummer-Strawn, L. (2005). Intention or experience? Predictors of continued breastfeeding. *Health Education & Behavior, 32*(2), 208-226. doi: 10.1177/1090198104271971.

Eidelman, A.I. (2012). Breastfeeding and the use of human milk: An analysis of the American academy of pediatrics 2012 breastfeeding policy statement. *Breastfeeding Medicine, 7*(5), 323-324. doi: 10.1089/bfm.2012.0067 [doi].

Fein, S.B., Labiner-Wolfe, J., Shealy, K.R., Li, R., Chen, J., & Grummer-Strawn, L.M. (2008). Infant feeding practices study II: Study methods. *Pediatrics. 122*(Suppl 2), S28-35. doi: 10.1542/peds.2008-1315c.

Horta, B.L., & Victora, C.G. (2013a). *Short-term effects of breastfeeding: A systematic review on the benefits of breastfeeding on diarrhoea and pneumonia mortality.* Geneva: World Health Organization.

Horta, B.L. & Victora, C.G. (2013b). *Long-term effects of breastfeeding: A systematic review on the benefits of breastfeeding on diarrhoea and pneumonia mortality.* Geneva: World Health Organization.

Meedya, S., Fahy, K., & Kable, A. (2010). Factors that positively influence breastfeeding duration to 6 months: A literature review. *Women & Birth, 23*(4), 135-145. doi: 10.1016/j.wombi.2010.02.002.

Nommsen-Rivers, L.A., & Dewey, K.G. (2009). Development and validation of the infant feeding intentions scale. *Maternal Child Health Journal, 13*(3), 334-342. doi: 10.1007/s10995-008-0356-y [doi].

Differences in Early Breastfeeding Experiences and Outcomes in Spanish versus English-Speaking Latinas from the Early Lactation Success Study Cohort of First-Time Mothers

Ahluwalia, I. B., D'Angelo, D., Morrow, B., & McDonald, J. A. (2012). Association between acculturation and breastfeeding among Hispanic women data from the Pregnancy Risk Assessment and Monitoring System. *Journal of Human Lactation, 28*(2), 167-173.

Centers for Disease Control and Prevention. (2007). *National Immunization Survey.* Retrieved from: http://www.cdc.gov/breastfeeding/data/NIS_data/2007/socio-demographic_formula.html

Chapman, D. J., & Pérez Escamilla, R. (2011). Acculturative type is associated with breastfeeding duration among low-income Latinas. *Maternal & Child Nutrition, 9*(2), 188-198.

Dennis, C. L. (2006). The breastfeeding self-efficacy scale: Psychometric assessment of the short form. *Journal of Obstetric, Gynecologic, & Neonatal Nursing, 32*(6), 734-744.

References

Guendelman, S., & Siega-Riz, A. M. (2002). Infant feeding practices and maternal dietary intake among Latino immigrants in California. *Journal of Immigrant Health,* 4(3), 137-146.

Li, R., Rock, V. J., & Grummer-Strawn, L. (2007). Changes in public attitudes toward breastfeeding in the United States, 1999-2003. *Journal of the American Dietetic Association,* 107(1), 122-127.

Nommsen-Rivers, L. A., Cohen, R. J., Chantry, C. J., & Dewey, K. G. (2010). The Infant Feeding Intentions scale demonstrates construct validity and comparability in quantifying maternal breastfeeding intentions across multiple ethnic groups. *Maternal & Child Nutrition,* 6(3), 220-227.

Passel, J. S., Cohn, D., & Lopez, M. H. (2011). *Hispanics account for more than half of nation's growth in past decade. Pew Hispanic Center.* Retrieved from: http://pewhispanic.org/files/reports/140.pdf

Singh, G. K., Kogan, M. D., & Dee, D. L. (2007). Nativity/immigrant status, race/ethnicity, and socioeconomic determinants of breastfeeding initiation and duration in the United States, 2003. *Pediatrics, 119*(Supplement 1), S38-S46.

Chapter 3

Brown Mamas Breastfeed—An Analysis of African American Women's Breastfeeding Experiences Shared through an Online Blog Project

Glauser, B., & Strauss, A. (1967). *The discovery of grounded theory: Strategies for qualitative research.* Piscataway, N.J.: Transaction Publishers.

Jeanine. (2011, June 28). *The Brown Mamas Breastfeed Project* [Web log comment]. Retrieved from http://itsbetterathome.wordpress.com/the-brown-mamas-breastfeed-project/

Ma, P., & Magnus, J. (2012). Exploring the concept of positive deviance related to breastfeeding initiation in black and white WIC enrolled first-time mothers. *Maternal and Child Health Journal, 16*(8), 1583-1593.

Sangodele-Ayoka, A. (2011, April 26). *The Brown Mamas Breastfeed Project.* Retrieved from: http://www.soulvegmama.com/page/brown-mamas-breastfeed-project/

Sweet, M., & Simon, M. (2009). As mass media evolves into "masses of media," what are the implications for our health? *Medical Journal of Australia, 191*(11/12), 618-619.

U.S. Department of Health and Human Services. (2010). *National Immunization Survey 2007*. Retrieved from: http://www.cdc.gov/breastfeeding/data/NIS_data/2007/socio-demographic_any.htm

West, J., Hall, P. C., Hanson, C., Thackeray, R., Barnes, M., Neiger, B., et al. (2011). Breastfeeding and blogging: Exploring the utility of blogs to promote breastfeeding. *American Journal of Health Education, 42*(2), 106-115.

Early Infant Feeding Practices among Mothers with High Body Mass Index

Fein, S.B., Labiner-Wolfe, J., Shealy, K.R., Li, R., Chen, J., & Grummer-Strawn, L.M. (2008). Infant feeding practices study II: Study methods. *Pediatrics, 122,* S28-S35.

Gaffney, K.F., Kitsantas, P., & Cheema, J. (2012). Clinical practice guidelines for feeding behaviors and weight-for-age at 12 months: A secondary analysis of the Infant Feeding Practices Study II. *Worldviews on Evidence-Based Nursing, 9*(4), 234-242.

Li, R., Fein, S.B., & Grummer-Strawn, L.M. (2008). Association of breastfeeding intensity and bottle-emptying behaviors at early infancy with infants' risk for excess weight at late infancy. *Pediatrics, 122,* S77-84.

Kitsantas, P., & Gaffney, K.F. (2010). Risk profiles for overweight/obesity among preschoolers. *Early Human Development, 86,* 563-568.

Ogden, C.L., Carrol, M.D., Curtin, L.R., Lamb, M.M., & Flegal, K.M. (2010). Prevalence of high body mass index in U.S. children and adolescents, 2007-2008. *Journal of American Medical Association, 303*(3), 242-249.

Rooney, B.L., Mathiason, M.A., & Schauberger, C.W. (2011). Predictors of obesity in childhood, adolescence, and adulthood in a birth cohort. *Maternal Child Health Journal, 15*, 1166-1175.

Seach, K.A., Dharmage, S.C., Lowe, A.J., & Dixon, J.B. (2010). Delayed introduction of solid feeding reduces child overweight and obesity at 10 years. *International Journal of Obesity, 34*, 1475-1479.

World Health Organization. (2008). *Childhood overweight and obesity.* Retrieved from: http://www.who.int/dietphysicalactivity/childhood/en/

Breastfeeding Narratives among WIC Participants in Alamance County, North Carolina

Cameron, B., Javanparast, S., Labbok, M., Scheckter, R., & McIntyre, E. (2012). Breastfeeding support in childcare: An international comparison of findings from Australia and the United States. *Breastfeeding Medicine, 7*, 163-166.

Chapman, D.J., Damio, G., Young, S., & Perez-Escamilla, R. (2004). Effectiveness of breastfeeding peer counseling in a low-income, predominately Latina population. *Archives of Pediatrics and Adolescent Medicine, 158*, 897-902.

References

Dykes, F. (2005). "Supply" and "demand": Breastfeeding as labour. *Social Science & Medicine, 60*, 2283-2293.

Evans, K., Labbok, M., & Abrahams, S.W. (2011). WIC and breastfeeding support services: Does the mix of services offered vary with race and ethnicity? *Breastfeeding Medicine, 6*, 401-406.

Fiedling, J.E., & Gilchick, R.A. (2011). Positioning for prevention from day 1 (and before). *Breastfeeding Medicine, 6*, 249-255

Knaak, S.J. (2010). Contextualising risk, constructing choice: Breastfeeding and good mothering in risk society. *Health, Risk, & Society 12*(4), 345-355.

Kronborg, H., & Kok, G. (2011). Development of a postnatal education program for breastfeeding mothers in community settings: Intervention mapping as a useful guide. *Journal of Human Lactation, 27*, 339-349.

Ma, P., & Magnus, J.H. (2012). Exploring the concept of positive deviance related to breastfeeding initiation in black and white WIC enrolled first time mothers. *Maternal Child Health Journal, 16*(8), 1583-1593.

Mitchell-Box, K., & Braun, K.L. (2012). Fathers' thoughts on breastfeeding and implications for a theory-based intervention. *Journal of Obstetric, Gynecologic, & Neonatal Nursing, 41*(6), E41-E50. doi: 10.1111/j.1552-6909.2012.01399.x.

Morrissey, S. (2010). Metaphors of relief: High risk pregnancy in a context of health policy for the "underserving" poor. *Human Organization, 69*(4), 352-361.

Quandt, S.A. (1995). Sociocultural aspects of the lactation process. In K. Dettwyler & P. Stuart-Macadam (Eds.), *Breastfeeding: Biocultural perspectives* (pp. 127-144). New York: Walter de Gruyter.

Shim, J.E., Kim, J., & Heiniger, J.B. (2012). Breastfeeding duration in relation to childcare arrangement and participation in the Special Supplemental Nutrition Program for Women, Infants, and Children. *Journal of Human Lactation, 28,* 28-35.

Singer, M. (1995). Beyond the ivory tower: Critical praxis in medical anthropology. *Medical Anthropology Quarterly, 9*(1), 80-106.

Stremler, J., & Lovera, D. (2004). Insight from a breastfeeding peer support pilot program for husbands and fathers of Texas WIC participants. *Journal of Human Lactation, 20,* 417-422.

Tenfelde, S., Finnegan, L., & Hill, P.D. (2011). Predictors of breastfeeding exclusivity in a WIC sample. *Journal of Obstetric, Gynecologic, & Neonatal Nursing, 40,* 179-189.

Walsh, E.G. (2012). Health disparities: Breastfeeding's role in closing the gap. *Breastfeeding Medicine, 7,* 1-2.

Wiley, A.S., & Allen, J.S. (2009). *Medical anthropology: A biocultural approach.* New York: Oxford University Press, Inc.

The Challenges of Nighttime Breastfeeding in the U.S.

American Academy of Pediatrics Task Force on Sudden Infant Death. (2005). The changing concept of Sudden Infant Death Syndrome: Diagnostic coding shifts, controversies regarding the sleeping environment, and new variables to consider in reducing risk. *Pediatrics, 116*(5), 1245-1255.

American Academy of Pediatrics Task Force on Sudden Infant Death Syndrome. (2011). SIDS and other sleep-related infant deaths: Expansion of recommendations for a safe infant sleeping environment. *Pediatrics, 128*(5), e1341-e1367.

Apple, R. D. (1987). *Mothers and medicine: A social history of infant feeding, 1890-1950.* Madison, WI.: University of Wisconsin Press.

Ball, H. L., & Volpe, L. E. (2013). SIDS risk reduction and infant sleep location: Moving the discussion forward. *Social Science and Medicine, 79*, 84-91.

Eidelman, A. I., & Gartner, L. M. (2006). Bedsharing with unimpaired parents is not an important risk for sudden infant death syndrome: To the editor. *Pediatrics, 117*(3), 991.

Gettler, L., & McKenna, J. (2010). Never sleep with baby? Or keep me close but keep me safe: Eliminating inappropriate safe infant sleep rhetoric in the United States. *Current Pediatric Reviews, 6*(1), 71-77.

Gottlieb, A. (2004). *The afterlife is where we come from: The culture of infancy in West Africa.* Chicago: University of Chicago Press.

Hausman, B., Smith, P. H., & Labbok, M. H. (2012). Introduction: Breastfeeding constraints and realities. In P. H. Smith, B. Hausman & M. H. Labbok (Eds.), *Beyond health, beyond choice: Breastfeeding constraints and realities* (pp. 1-11). New Brunswick, NJ: Rutgers University Press.

Hausman, B. L. (2003). *Mother's milk: Breastfeeding controversies in American culture.* New York: Routledge.

Hausman, B. L. (2011). *Viral mothers: Breastfeeding in the age of HIV/AIDS.* Ann Arbor, MI: University of Michigan Press.

Jenni, O. G., & O'Connor, B. B. (2005). Children's sleep: An interplay between culture and biology. *Pediatrics, 115*(1), 204-216.

Kendall-Tackett, K., Cong, Z., & Hale, T. W. (2010). Mother-infant sleep locations and nighttime feeding behavior. *Clinical Lactation, 1,* 27-31.

References

McKenna, J. J., Ball, H. L., & Gettler, L. T. (2007). Mother-infant cosleeping, breastfeeding and Sudden Infant Death Syndrome: What biological anthropology has discovered about normal infant sleep and pediatric sleep medicine. *American Journal of Physical Anthropology* (Supplement 45), 134(S45), 133-161.

McKenna, J. J., & McDade, T. (2005). Why babies should never sleep alone: A review of the co-sleeping controversy in relation to SIDS, bedsharing, and breast feeding. *Paediatric Respiratory Reviews, 6*(2), 134-152.

Morelli, G. A., Rogoff, B., Oppenheim, D., & Goldsmith, D. (1992). Cultural variation in infants' sleeping arrangements: Questions of independence. *Developmental Psychology, 28*(4), 604-613.

Shweder, R. A., Jensen, L. A., & Goldstein, W. (1995). Who sleeps by whom revisited: A method for extracting the moral goods implicit in practice. *New Directions for Child Development, 67*, 21-39.

Stearns, P. N., Rowland, P., & Giarnella, L. (1996). Children's sleep: Sketching historical change. *Journal of Social History, 30*(2), 345-366.

Tomori, C. (2014). *Nighttime breastfeeding: An American cultural dilemma.* New York: Berghahn Books.

Wolf, J. H. (2001). *Don't kill your baby: Public health and the decline of breastfeeding in the nineteenth and twentieth centuries*. Columbus, OH: Ohio State University Press.

The Challenge of Late Preterm Birth on Realizing Breastfeeding Intentions

Ayton, J., Hansen, E., Quinn, S., & Nelson, M. (2012). Factors associated with initiation and exclusive breastfeeding at hospital discharge: Late preterm compared to 37 week gestation mother and infant cohort. *International Breastfeeding Journal, 7*(1), 16. doi: 10.1186/1746-4358-7-16.

Brandon, D. H., Tully, K. P., Silva, S., Thompson, J., Malcolm, W., Murtha, A., Turner, B., & Holditch-Davis, D. (2011). Emotional responses of mothers of late-preterm and term infants. *Journal of Obstetric, Gynecologic, and Neonatal Nursing, 40*(6), 719-731. doi: 10.1111/j.1552-6909.2011.01290.x

Centers for Disease Control and Prevention (CDC). (2013). Progress in increasing breastfeeding and reducing racial/ethnic differences—United States, 2000–2008 births. *Morbidity and Mortality Weekly Report, 62*(5), 77-80. Retrieved from: http://www.cdc.gov/mmwr/preview/mmwrhtml/mm6205a1.htm

Demirci, J. D., Sereika, S. M., & Bogen, D. (2013). Prevalence and predictors of early breastfeeding among late preterm mother-infant dyads. *Breastfeeding Medicine, 8*(3), 277-285. doi: 10.1089/bfm.2012.0075.

References

Liu, P., Qiao, L., Xu, F., Zhang, M., Wang, Y., & Binns, C. W. (2013). Factors associated with breastfeeding duration: A 30-month cohort study in Northwest China. *Journal of Human Lactation, 29*(2), 253-259. doi: 10.1177/0890334413477240.

Martin, J. A., Hamilton, B. E., Osterman, M. J. K., Curtin, S. C., & Mathews, T. J. (2013). Births: Final data for 2012. *National Vital Statistics Reports, 62*(9). Retrieved from: http://www.cdc.gov/nchs/data/nvsr/nvsr62/nvsr62_09.pdf

Meier, P. P. (2010). *Breastfeeding your late preterm infant.* McHenry, IL: Medela, Inc.

Meier, P., Patel, A. L., Wright, K., & Engstrom, J. L. (2013). Management of breastfeeding during and after the maternity hospitalization for late preterm infants. *Clinics in Perinatology, 40*(4), 689-705. doi: 10.1016/j.clp.2013.07.014.

Miles, M. B., Huberman, A. M., & Saldana, J. (2013). *Qualitative data analysis: An expanded sourcebook, 2nd Ed.* Thousand Oaks, CA: Sage.

Nommsen-Rivers, L. A., Chantry, C. J., Cohen, R. J., & Dewey, K.G. (2010). Comfort with the idea of formula feeding helps explain ethnic disparity in breastfeeding intentions among expectant first-time mothers. *Breastfeeding Medicine, 5*(1), 25-33. doi: 10.1089/bfm.2009.0052.

Nommsen-Rivers, L. A., & Dewey, K. G. (2009). Development and validation of the infant feeding intentions scale. *Maternal and Child Health Journal, 13*(3), 334-342. doi: 10.1007/s10995-008-0356-y.

Radtke, J. V. (2011). The paradox of breastfeeding-associated morbidity among late preterm infants. *Journal of Obstetric, Gynecologic, and Neonatal Nursing, 40*(1), 9-24. doi: 10.1111/j.1552-6909.2010.01211.x.

Wang, M.L., Dorer, D.J., Fleming, M.P., & Catlin, E.A. (2004). Clinical outcomes of near-term infants. *Pediatrics, 114*(2), 372-376.

Updegrove, K. (2013). Nonprofit human milk banking in the United States. *Journal of Midwifery and Women's Health*, [e-pub ahead of print] doi: 10.1111/j.1542-2011.2012.00267.x.

Zanardo, V., Gambina, I., Begley, C., Litta, P., Cosmi, E., Giustardi, A., & Trevisanuto, D. (2011). Psychological distress and early lactation performance of mothers of preterm infants. *Early Human Development, 87*(4), 321-323. doi:10.1016/j.earlhumdev.2011.01.035.

Expectant Moms Respond to "Risk" and "Benefit" Language in Breastfeeding Promotion: Evaluating the Impact of Language on Efficacy

References

Heinig, M. J. (2009). Are there risks to using risk-based messages to promote breastfeeding? *Journal of Human Lactation, 25,* 7–8.

Kelleher, C. M. (2006). The physical challenges of early breastfeeding. *Social Science and Medicine, 63,* 2727–2738.

Kukla, R. (2006). Ethics and ideology in breastfeeding advocacy campaigns. *Hypatia, 21,* 157–80.

Labbok, M. H. (1999). Health sequelae of breastfeeding for the mother. *Clinics in Perinatology, 6,* 491–503.

MacNiel, M. E., Labbok, M. H., & Abrahams, S.W. (2010). What are the risks associated with formula feeding? A re-analysis and review. *Birth, 37,* 50–58.

Merewood, A., & Heinig, J. (2004). Efforts to promote breastfeeding in the United States: Development of a national breastfeeding awareness campaign. *Journal of Human Lactation, 20,* 140–145.

Nommsen–Rivers, L. A., Chantry, C. J., Cohen, R. J., & Dewey, K. G. (2010). Comfort with the idea of formula-feeding helps explain ethnic disparity in breastfeeding intentions among expectant first-time mothers. *Breastfeeding Medicine, 5,* 25–33.

Slaw, R. (1999). *1999 LLLI conference sessions: Promoting breastfeeding or promoting guilt?* Retrieved from: http://llli.org/NB/NBSepOct99p171.html

Smith, J., Dunstone, M., & Elliott-Rudder, M. (2009). Health professional knowledge of breastfeeding: Are the health risks of infant formula-feeding accurately conveyed by the titles and abstracts of journal articles? *Journal of Human Lactation, 25*, 350–358.

Taylor, E., & Wallace, L.E. (2012). For shame: Feminism, breastfeeding advocacy, and maternal guilt. *Hypatia, 27*, 76-98.

Wallace, L. E., & Taylor, E. (2011). Potential risks of "risk" language in breastfeeding advocacy. *Women and Health, 51*(4), 299-320.

Wiessinger, D. (1996). Watch your language! The language of breastfeeding. *Journal of Human Lactation, 12*, 1–4.

Wolf, J. B. (2007). Is breast really best? Risk and total motherhood in the national breastfeeding awareness campaign. *Journal of Health Politics, Policy and Law, 32*, 595–636.

Chapter 4

Advancing the Breastfeeding-Friendly Campus: Cultivating University Climates can Inspire Change in the Community

Saxon, A. (2012). *The lactating body on display: Collective rhetoric and resistant discourse in breastfeeding activism.* English theses. Paper 125.

References

Development of Indicators to Evaluate the Presence of Worksite Breastfeeding Supportive Policies, Benefits, and Environments

Bureau of Labor Statistics. (2009). *Women in the labor force: A databook*. Retrieved from: http://www.bls.gov/cps/wlf-intro-2009.htm

Office of Disease Prevention and Health Promotion. (2009). *Developing healthy people 2020: The road ahead*. Washington, DC: United States Department of Health and Human Services.

Shealy, K. R., Li, R., Benton-Davis, S., & Grummer-Strawn, L. M. (2005). *The CDC guide to breastfeeding interventions*. Atlanta: Centers for Disease Control and Prevention.

United States Department of Labor. (2008). *Labor force participation of mothers with infants in 2008*. Retrieved from: http://www.bls.gov/opub/ted/2009/may/wk4/art04.htm

United States Department of Health and Human Services. (2008). *The business case for breastfeeding*. Bethesda, MD: United States Department of Health and Human Services.

United States Department of Health and Human Services. (2011). *The Surgeon General's Call to Action to Support Breastfeeding*. Washington, DC: United States Department of Health and Human Services, Offices of the Surgeon General.

Establishing an Employee Lactation Program in a Large Municipal Health Agency.

United States Department of Health and Human Services. (2008). *The business case for breastfeeding*. Bethesda, MD: United States Department of Health and Human Services.

Chapter 5

Evaluation of Breastfeeding Peer Support in a Rural Area: What Works for Young, Disadvantaged Women and Their Babies?

Alexander, J., Anderson, T., Grant, M., Sanghera, J., & Jackson, D. (2003). An evaluation of a support group for breastfeeding women in Salisbury, UK. *Midwifery, 19*(3), 215-220.

Condon, L., & Ingram, J. (2011). Increasing support for breastfeeding: What can children's centres do? *Health and Social Care in the Community, 19*(6), 617-625.

References

Dykes, F. (2005). Government funded breastfeeding peer support projects: Implications forpractice. *Maternal and Child Nutrition, 1*, 21-31.

Dowling, S., & Evans, D. (2013). *Breastfeeding peer support in Wiltshire: An evaluation*. Project Report. University of the West of England. Retrieved from: http://eprints.uwe.ac.uk/21983/

Hoddinott, P., Lee, A.J., & Pill, R. (2006). Effectiveness of a breastfeeding peer support coaching intervention in rural Scotland. *Birth, 33*(1), 27-36.

Ingram, J., Rosser, J., & Jackson, D. (2004). Breastfeeding peer supports and a community support group: Evaluating their effectiveness. *Maternal and Child Nutrition, 1*, 111-118.

Ingram, L., MacArthur, C., Khan, K., Deeks, J.J., & Jolly, K. (2010). Effect of antenatal peer support on breastfeeding initiation: A systematic review. *Canadian Medical Association Journal, 182*(16), 1739-1746.

Jolly, K., Ingram, L., Freemantle, N., Khan, K., Chambers, J., Hamburger, R., Brown, J., Dennis, C-L., & MacArthur, C. (2012). Effect of a peer support service on breastfeeding continuation in the UK: A randomised controlled trial. *Midwifery, 28*, 740-745.

Kaunonen, M., Hannula, L., & Tarkka, M-T. (2012). A systematic review of peer support interventionsfor breastfeeding. *Journal of Clinical Nursing, 21,* 1943-1954.

National Institute for Health and Clinical Excellence. (2008). *A peer-support programme forwomen who breastfeed: Commissioning guide, implementing NICE guidance.* Retrieved from: http://www.gserve.nice.org.uk/media/63D/7B/BreastfeedingCommissioningGuide.pdf

Pawson, R. (2013). *The science of evaluation: A realist manifesto.* London: Sage.

Pawson, R. (2006). *Evidence-based policy: A realist perspective.* London: Sage.

Pawson, R., & Tilly, N. (1997). *Realistic evaluation.* London: Sage.

Phipps, B. (2006). Peer support for breastfeeding in the UK. *British Journal of General Practice, 56*(524), 166-167.

Wade, D., Halning, S., & Day, A. (2009). Breastfeeding peer support: Are there additional benefits? *Community Practitioner, 82*(12), 30-33.

World Health Organization. (2003). *Community-based strategies for breastfeeding promotion and support in developing countries.* Retrieved from: http://whqlibdoc.who.int/publications/2003/9241591218.pdf

From Bottles to Breasts in Rural Haiti

Berggren, W., Simeon, F., Berggren, G., & Tobing, S. (1998). *Program evaluation Haitian Health Foundation. USAID, 56.* www.haitianhealthfoundation.org

Sabanda-Mulder, F. S. (Jun. 1995). *Informations Generales. Campagne nationale de la promotion, la protection, et l'appui a l'allaitement maternel en Haiti.* Port-au-Prince, Haiti: UNICEF.

Associations between Frequency of Interpersonal Contact Opportunities and Exclusive Breastfeeding Coverage in USAID's Child Survival and Health Grants Program

Britton, C., McCormick, F.M., Renfrew, M.J., Wade, A., & King, S.E. (2007). Support for breastfeeding mothers. *Cochrane Database of Systematic Reviews, (1)*, CD00114.

Davis, T.P., Wetzel, C., Hernandez Avilan, E., de Mendoza Lopes, C., Chase, R.P., Winch, P.J., & Perry, H.B. (2013). Reducing child global undernutrition at scale in Sofala Province, Mozambique, using care group volunteers to communicate health messages to mothers. *Global Health Science and Practice, 1*(1), 35-51. doi: 10.9745/GHSP-D-12-00045.

Green, C. (1999). *Improving breastfeeding behaviors: Evidence from two decades of intervention research. LINKAGES Project.* Retrieved from: http://pdf.usaid.gov/pdf_docs/PNACH559.

Labbok, M. (2012). *Community interventions to promote optimal breastfeeding: Evidence on early initiation, any breastfeeding, exclusive breastfeeding, and continued breastfeeding. Infant and Young Child Nutrition (IYCN) Project.* Retrieved from: http://iycn.wpengine.netdna-cdn.com/files/IYCN_Literature_Review_Community_Breastfeeding_Interventions_Feb_121.pdf

Laughlin, M (2004). *The care group difference: A guide to mobilizing community-based volunteer health educators.* Retrieved from: http://www.mchip.net/sites/default/files/Care_Group_Manual_ENGLISH.pdf

McNulty, J. (2005). *Positive deviance/hearth essential elements: A resource guide for sustainably rehabilitating malnourished children (addendum).* Washington, D.C.: CORE Group. Retrieved from: http://www.positivedeviance.org/pdf/manuals/addendum.pdf

Renfrew, M.J., McCormick, F.M., Wade, A., Quinn, B., & Dowswell, T. (2012). Support for healthy breastfeeding mothers with healthy term babies. *Cochrane Database of Systematic Reviews,* (5): CD001141. doi: 10.1002/14651858.CD001141.pub4

References

Yourkavitch, J., & Lutz, E. (2010). *How women-centered approaches contribute to an increase in exclusive breastfeeding around the world.* Presented at the Fifth Symposium for Breastfeeding and Feminism, Greensboro, NC.

Chapter 6

Lactation Consulting and the Role of Family-Centered Care in Professional Breastfeeding Support

American Academy of Pediatrics. (2012). Patient- and family-centered care and the pediatrician's role. *Pediatrics, 129*(2), 394-404. doi: 10.1542/peds.2011-3084

Corlett, J., & Twycross, A. (2006). Negotiation of parental roles within family-centred care: A review of the research. *Journal of Clinical Nursing, 15*(10), 1308-1316. doi: 10.1111/j.1365-2702.2006.01407.x

Gramling, L., Hickman, K., & Bennett, S. (2004). What makes a good family-centered partnership between women and their practitioners? A qualitative study. Birth, 31(1), 43-48.

International Board of Lactation Consultant Examiners. (2008). *Scope of practice for International Board Certified Lactation Consultants.* Retrieved from: http://iblce.org/upload/downloads/ScopeOfPractice.pdf

Johnson, B. H. (2000). Family-centered care: Four decades of progress. *Families, Systems, and Health, 18*(2), 137-156.

Kuo, D. Z., Houtrow, A. J., Arango, P., Kuhlthau, K. A., Simmons, J. M., & Neff, J. M. (2012). Family-centered care: Current applications and future directions in pediatric health care. *Maternal and Child Health Journal, 16*(2), 297-305. doi: 10.1007/s10995-011-0751-7

MacKean, G. L., Thurston, W. E., & Scott, C. M. (2005). Bridging the divide between families and health professionals' perspectives on family-centred care. *Health Expectations, 8*(1), 74-85. doi: 10.1111/j.1369-7625.2005.00319.x.

Maternal and Child Health Bureau. (2005). *Definition of family-centered care.* Retrieved from: http://www.familyvoices.org/admin/work_family_centered/files/FCCare.pdf

Pettoello-Mantovani, M., Campanozzi, A., Maiuri, L., & Giardino, I. (2009). Family-oriented and family-centered care in pediatrics. *Italian Journal of Pediatrics, 35*(1), 12. doi: 10.1186/1824-7288-35-12.

Pillitteri, A. (2007). *Maternal and child health nursing: Care of the childbearing and childrearing family.* Retrieved from: http://downloads.lww.com/wolterskluwer_vitalstream_com/sample-content/9780781777766_Pillitteri/samples/Chapter01.pdf.

References

U.S. Department of Health and Human Services. (2011). *The Surgeon General's Call to Action to Support Breastfeeding.* Washington, DC: U.S. Department of Health and Human Services, Office of the Surgeon General.

Application of the Relational Theory to an Academic Program in Maternal Child Health Lactation Consulting: The Transformative Power of Learning

Belenky, M.F., Clinchy, B.M., Goldberger, N.R., & Tarule, J.M. (1986). *Women's ways of knowing: The development of self, voice and mind.* New York: Basic Books.

Hayes, E., & Flannery, D. (2000). *Women as learners: The significance of gender in adult learning.* San Francisco: Jossey-Bass.

Mezirow, J. (2012). Learning to thing like an adult. In E.W. Taylor & P. Cranton (Eds.), *The handbook of transformative learning: Theory, research and practice.* San Francisco: Jossey-Bass.

Rew, L. (2008). Self-reflection. In B.M. Dossey & L.Keegan (Eds.) *Holistic nursing: A handbook for practice.* Sudbury, MA: Jones and Bartlett.

Ruddick, S. (1995). *Maternal thinking: Toward a politics of peace.* Boston MA: Beacon Hill Press.

Stanton, A. (1997). Reconfiguring teaching and knowing in the college classroom. In N.R. Goldberger, J. Turule, B. Clinchy, & M.F. Belenky (Eds.), *Women's ways of knowing: The development of self, voice and mind*. New York: Basic Books.

Taylor, E.W., & Cranton, P. (Eds.) (2012). *The handbook of transformative learning: Theory, research and practice*. San Francisco: Jossey-Bass.

Low-Income Women's Experiences with Breastfeeding and Lactation Support: A Program Evaluation of a Community Home Visitation Service

Buckley, K. (2009). A double-edged sword: Lactation consultants' perceptions of the impact of breast pumps on the practice of breastfeeding. *Journal of Perinatal Education, 18*(2),13-22.

Centers for Disease Control and Prevention. (2010). *Breastfeeding among U.S. children born 1999–2007*. CDC National Immunization Survey. Retrieved from: http://www.cdc.gov/breastfeeding/data/NIS_data/index.htm

Gross, S. M., Resnik, A.K., Nanda, J.P., Cross-Barnet, C., Augustyn, M., Kelly, L., & Paige, D.M. (2011). Early postpartum: A critical period in setting the path for breastfeeding success. *Breastfeeding Medicine, 6*, 407-412.

Hannula, L., Kaunonen, M., & Tarkka, M.T. (2008). A systematic review of professional support interventions for breastfeeding. *Journal of Clinical Nursing, 17*(9), 1132-1143.

Hausman, B. L. (2012). Feminism and breastfeeding: Rhetoric, ideology, and the material realities of women's lives. In P.H. Smith, M. Labbok, and B. Hausman (Eds.), *Beyond health, beyond choice: Breastfeeding constraints and realities*. New Brunswick, NJ: Rutgers University Press.

Mannan, I., Rahman, S.M., Sania, A., Seraji, H.R., Arifeen, S.E.,Winch, P.J., Darmstadt, G.L., Baqui, A., & Bangladesh Projahnmo Study Group. (2008). Can early postpartum home visits by trained community health workers improve breastfeeding of newborns? *Journal of Perinatology, 28*(9), 632-640.

McKeever, P., Slevens, B., Miller, K.L., MacDonell, J.W., Gibbins, S., Guerriere, D., Dunn, M.S., & Coyle, P.C. (2002). Home versus hospital breastfeeding support for newborns: A randomized controlled trial. *Birth, 29*(4), 258-265.

Ryan, A. S., Wenjun, Z., & Acosta, A. (2002). Breastfeeding continues to increase into the new millennium. *Pediatrics, 110*, 1103-1109.

Torres, J. (2009). *Pumps and scales: The medicalization of breastfeeding and the ideology of insufficient milk*. Presentation at the Annual Meeting of the American Sociological Association. San Francisco, CA.

U.S. Department of Health and Human Services. (2011). *The Surgeon General's Call to Action to Support Breastfeeding*. U.S. Department of Health and Human Services, Office of the Surgeon General.

"We Just Have This One Breastfeeding Brochure" (Sponsored by Enfamil): Exploring Breastfeeding Resources and Agenda-Setting in Pediatrics' Offices, WIC, LLL, and the Community Hospital

Ahluwalia, I. B., Tessaro, I., Grummer-Strawn, L.M., MacGowan, C., & Benton-Davis, S. (2000). Georgia's breastfeeding promotion program for low-income women. *Pediatrics, 105*(6), e85.

Bodribb, W. (2011). Barriers to translating evidence-based breastfeeding information into practice. Acta Paediatrica, 100, 486-490.

Centers for Disease Control and Prevention. (2012). *Breastfeeding report card, United States 2012: Outcome indicators. Based on the United States National Immunization Survey, 2009 Births*. Centers for Disease Control and Prevention, Department of Health and Human Services. Retrieved from: http://www.cdc.gov/breastfeeding/data/reportcard2.htm.

References

Cities by Population: Murfreesboro, TN. (2012). *City-data.com*. Retrieved from: http://www.city-data.com/city/Murfreesboro-Tennessee.html

Grawey, A. E., Marinelli, K. A., & Holmes, A. V. (2013). ABM Clinical Protocol# 14: Breastfeeding-friendly physician's office: Optimizing care for infants and children. Revised 2013. *Breastfeeding Medicine, 8*(2), 237-242.

Humphreys, A. S., Thompson, N. J., & Miner, K. R. (1998). Intention to breastfeed in low-income pregnant women: The role of social support and previous experience. *Birth. 25*(3), 169-174.

Kaufman, L., Deenadayalan, S., & Karpati, A. (2010). Breastfeeding ambivalence among low-income African American and Puerto Rican women in North and Central Brooklyn. *Maternal Child Health Journal, 14*(5), 696-704.

McCombs, M. E., & Shaw, D. L. (1972). The agenda-setting function of mass media. *Public Opinion Quarterly, 36*(2), 176-187.

Murfreesboro, TN Poverty Rate Data. (2012). *City-data.com*. Retrieved from: http://www.city-data.com/poverty/poverty-Murfreesboro-Tennessee.html

Persad, M. D., & Mensinger, J. L. (2008). Maternal breastfeeding attitudes: Association with breastfeeding intent and socio-demographics among urban primiparas. *Journal of Community Health, 33*, 53-60.

Shoemaker, P. J., & Vos, T. (2009). Gatekeeping theory. London: Routledge.Tennessee. (2009). *Percentage of children ever breastfed by age and exclusivity among children born in 2009. Kaiser family state health facts.* Retrieved from: http://www.statehealthfacts.org/profileind.jsp?rgn=44&ind=501

Growing Breastfeeding Advocates among the Next Generation of Nurses

Bozzette, M., & Posner, T. (2012). *Increasing student nurses' knowledge of breastfeeding in baccalaureate education. Nurse Education in Practice.* Retrieved from: http://dx.doi.org/10.1016/j.nepr.2012.08.013

Dodgson, J. E., & Tarrant, M. (2007). Outcomes of a breastfeeding educational intervention for baccalaureate nursing students. *Nurse Education Today, 27,* 856-867.

International Breastfeeding Centre. (2012). *Video clips.* Retrieved from: http://www.nbci.ca/index.php?option=com_content&view=category&layout=blog&id=6&Itemid=13

McKenna, L. (2003). Nurturing the future of midwifery through mentoring. *Australian Journal of Midwifery, 16*(2), 7-10.

References

Renfrew, M. J., Dyson, L., & Wallace, L. (2005). *The effectiveness of public health interventions to promote the duration of breastfeeding.* A systematic review. London: National Institute for Health and Clinical Excellence.

Spatz, D. L. (2005). The breastfeeding case study: A model for educating nursing students. *Journal of Nursing Education, 44*(9), 432-434.

Woolley, N. N., & Jarvis, Y. (2007). Situated cognition and cognitive apprenticeship: A model for teaching and learning clinical skills in a technologically rich and authentic learning environment. *Nurse Education Today, 27,* 73-79.

The Role of Growth Pattern Interpretations on U.S. Women's

American Academy of Pediatrics (AAP) Section on Breastfeeding. (2012). Breastfeeding and the use of human milk. *Pediatrics, 129*(3), e827-e841.

Behague, D. (1993). Growth monitoring and the promotion of breastfeeding. *Social Science & Medicine, 37*(12), 1565-1578.

Centers for Disease Control and Prevention (CDC). (2010). Use of World Health Organization and CDC growth charts for children aged 0-59 months in the United States. *Morbidity and Mortality Weekly Reports.* http://www.cdc.gov/mmwr/preview/mmwrhtml/rr5909a1.htm

De Onis, M., Garza, C., & Habicht, J.P. (1997). Time for a new growth reference. *Pediatrics, 100*(5), E8.

De Onis , M., Garza, C., Onyango, A.W., & Rolland-Cachera, M.F. (2009). WHO growth standards for infants and young children. *Archives of Pediatrics, 16,* 47-53.

De Jager, M., Hartley, K., Terrazas, J., & Merrill, J. (2012). Barriers to breastfeeding—A global survey on why women start and stop breastfeeding. *European Obstetrics and Gynaecology, 7*(Suppl.1), 25-30.

Dewey, K.G. (1998). Growth characteristics of breast-fed compared to formula-fed infants. *Biology of the Neonate, 74*(2), 94-105.

Dykes F., & Williams C. (1999). Falling by the wayside: A phenomenological exploration of perceived breast-milk inadequacy in lactating women. *Midwifery, 15*(4), 232-246.

References

Greer, F., & Bhatia, J.S. (2010). *CDC: Use WHO growth charts for children under 2. AAP News*. Retrieved from: www.aapnews.aappublications.org/content/31/11/1.1.full 31.

Heinig, M. J., Follett, J. R., Ishii, K. D., Kavanagh-Prochaska, K., Cohen, R., & Panchula, J. (2006). Barriers to compliance with infant-feeding recommendations among low-income women. *Journal of Human Lactation, 22*(1), 27-38.

Kramer, M.S., Guo, T., Platt, R.W., Vanilovich, I., Sevkovskaya, Z., Dzikovich, I., . . . Promotion of Breastfeeding Intervention Trials Study Group. (2004). Feeding effects on growth during infancy. *Journal of Pediatrics, 145*(5), 600-605.

Mei, Z., Odgen, C., Flegal, K.M., & Grummer-Strawn, L.M. (2008). Comparison of the prevalence of shortness, underweight, and overweight among U.S. children aged 0 to 59 months by using the CDC 2000 and the WHO 2006 growth charts. *Journal of Pediatrics, 153*(5), 622-628.

Panpanich R., Garner P., & Logan S. (2000). Is routine growth monitoring effective? A systematic review of trials. *Archives of Diseases of Childhood, 82*, 197-201.

Powers, N. G. (1999). Slow weight gain and low milk supply in the breastfeeding dyad. *Clinics in Perinatology, 26*(2), 399-430.

It Takes a Village

Sachs, M., Dykes, F., & Carter, B. (2006). Feeding by numbers: An ethnographic study of how breastfeeding women understand their babies' weight charts. *International Breastfeeding Journal, 22*; 1(29).

United States. Dept. of Health and Human Services. (2011). *The Surgeon General's Call to Action to Support Breastfeeding*. Washington, D.C.: Dept. of Health and Human Services, Office of the Surgeon General.

Walker, M. (2011). Beyond the initial 48-72 hours: Infant challenges. *Breastfeeding management for the clinician: Using the evidence*. Sudbury, MA: Jones and Bartlett.

World Health Organization. (2008). *WHO child growth standards*. Geneva: World Health Organization.

The Role of Postnatal Unit Bassinet Types on Enabling Early Breastfeeding

Ball, H. L. (2008). Evolutionary paediatrics: A case study in applying Darwinian medicine. In S. Elton & P. O'Higgins (Eds.), *Medicine and evolution: Current applications, future prospects* (pp. 127-152). London: CRC Press.

Ball, H.L., Ward-Platt, M.P., Heslop, E., Leech, S.J., & Brown, K.A. (2006). Randomised trial of infant sleep location on the postnatal ward. *Archives of Diseases of Childhood, 91*(12), 1005-1010.

References

Bartington S., Griffiths, L.J., Tate, A. R., & Dezateux, C. (2006). Are breastfeeding rates higher among mothers delivering in Baby-Friendly accredited maternity units in the UK? *International Journal of Epidemiology, 35*(5), 1178–1186. doi: 10.1093/ije/dyl155

Cramton, R., Zain-Ul-Abideen, M., & Whalen, B. (2009). Optimizing successful breastfeeding in the newborn. *Current Opinion in Pediatrics, 21*(3), 386-396. doi: 10.1097/MOP.0b013e32832b325a.

Forrester-Knauss, C., Merten, S., Weiss, C., Ackermann-Liebrich, U., & Zemp Stutz, E. (2013).The Baby-Friendly Hospital Initiative in Switzerland: Trends over a 9-year period. *Journal of Human Lactation, 29*(4), 510-516. doi: 10.1177/0890334413483923

McKenna, J. J., Mosko, S. S., & Richard, C. A. (1997). Bedsharing promotes breastfeeding. *Pediatrics, 100*(2 Pt 1), 214-219. doi: 10.1542/peds.100.2.214

Merten S., Dratva J., & Ackermann-Liebrich U. (2005). Do baby-friendly hospitals influence breastfeeding duration on a national level? *Pediatrics, 116*(5), e702–e708. doi:10.1542/peds.2005-0537

Odent, M. (2003). *Birth and breastfeeding: Rediscovering the needs of women during pregnancy and childbirth.* Forest Row, England: Clairview.

Philipp, B. L., Merewood, A., Miller, L. W., Chawla, N., Murphy-Smith, M. M., Gomes, J. S., Cimo, S., & Cook, J. T. (2001). Baby-Friendly Hospital Initiative improves breastfeeding initiation rates in a U.S. hospital setting. *Pediatrics, 108*(3), 677-681. doi: 10.1542/peds.108.3.677

Quandt, S. A. (1981). *The biobehavioral dynamics of the infant feeding process.* Doctor of Philosophy thesis, Michigan State University.

Tully, K. P., & Ball, H. L. (2012). Postnatal unit bassinet types when rooming-in after cesarean birth: Implications for breastfeeding and infant safety. *Journal of Human Lactation, 28*(4), 495-505. doi: 10.1177/0890334412452932

Wilkinson, S. (2004). Focus group research. In D. Silverman (Ed.). *Qualitative research: Theory, method, and practice* (2nd Ed.) (177-199). London: Sage Publications.

World Health Organization. (2006). *Pregnancy, childbirth, postpartum and newborn care: A guide for essential practice.* Geneva: World Health Organization. Retrieved from: http://www.who.int/reproductivehealth/publications/maternal_perinatal_health/924159084X/en/index.html

World Health Organization (2009). *Acceptable medical reasons for breast-milk substitutes.* World Health Organization: Geneva. Retrieved from: http://www.who.int/maternal_child_adolescent/documents/WHO_FCH_CAH_09.01/en/

Yamauchi, Y., & Yamanouchi, I. (1990). The relationship between rooming-in/not rooming-in and breastfeeding variables. *Acta Pædiatrica, 79*(11), 1017-1022. doi: 10.1111/j.1651-2227.1990.tb11377.x

Chapter 7

Increasing the Use of Donor Human Milk: An Assessment of Knowledge, Beliefs, and Practices Among Key Stakeholders in North Carolina

Cohen, R. (2007). Current issues in human milk banking. *Neos Review, 8*(7), 289-295.

Dunn, L. (2012). *2012 update on donor milk banking* [PowerPoint slides]. Rex Hospital. Raleigh, NC. Retrieved in person.

Human Milk Banking Association of North America. (2012). *HMBANA milk bank locations*. Retrieved from: https://www.hmbana.org/milk-bank-locations

Human Milk Banking Association of North America. (2013). *Processing.* Retrieved from: https://www.hmbana.org/processing

Lucas, A., & Cole, T.J. (1990). Breast milk and neonatal necrotizing enterocolitis. *Lancet, 336,* 1519-1523.

U.S. Department of Health and Human Services. (2011). *The Surgeon General's Call to Action to Support Breastfeeding.* Retrieved from: http://www.surgeongeneral.gov/topics/breastfeeding/calltoactiontosupportbreastfeeding.pdf.

World Health Organization. (2011). *Feeding of low-birthweight infants.* Retrieved from: http://www.who.int/elena/titles/supplementary_feeding/en/index.html.

The Gift of Milk: How Altruistic Milk Sharing Practices Empower Women

Akre, J. E., Gribble, K. D., & Minchin, M. (2011). Milk sharing: From private practice to public pursuit. *International Breastfeeding Journal, 6*(8), 1-3.

Geraghty, S. R., Heier, J. E., & Rasmussen, K. M. (2011). Got milk? Sharing human milk via the Internet. *Public Health Reports, 126,* 161-164.

Geraghty, S. R., McNamara, K. A., Dillon, C. E., Hogan, J. S., Kwiek, J. J., & Keim, S. A. (2013). Buying human milk via the internet: Just a click away. *Breastfeeding Medicine, 8*(6), 474-478. doi: 10.1089/bfm.2013.0048

Gribble, K. (2013). Peer-to-peer milk donors' and recipients' experiences and perceptions of donor milk banks. *JOGNN, 42*(4), 451-461.

References

Gribble, K. D., & Hausman, B. L. (2012). Milk sharing and formula feeding: Infant feeding risks in comparative perspective. *Australasian Medical Journal, 5*(5), 275-283.

Hausman, B. L. (2006). Contamination and contagion: Environmental toxins, HIV/AIDS, and the problem of the maternal body. *Hypatia, 21*(1), 137-156. doi: 10.1111/j.1527-2001.2006.tb00969.x

Keim, S. A., Hogan, J. S., McNamara, K. A., Gudimetla, V., Dillon, C. E., Kwiek, J. J., & Geraghty, S. R. (2013). Microbial contamination of human milk purchased via the internet. *Pediatrics, 132*(5), e1227-e1235. doi: 10.1542/peds.2013-1687

Shaw, R., & Bartlett, A. (2010). *Giving breast milk: Body ethics and contemporary breastfeeding practice.* Bradford, Ontario: Demeter Press.

Updegrove, K. H. (2013a). Donor human milk banking: Growth, challenges, and the role of HMBANA. *Breastfeeding Medicine, 8,* 435-437. doi: 10.1089/bfm.2013.0079

Updegrove, K. H. (2013b). Nonprofit human milk banking in the United States. *Journal of Midwifery and Women's Health, 58*(5), 1542-2011.

Donor Human Milk: Past, Present and Future

AAP Working Group on Breastfeeding. (1997). Breastfeeding and the use of human milk. *Pediatrics, 100*(6), 1035-1039.

ADA. (2011). *Infant feedings: Guidelines for preparation of human milk and formula in health care facilities, Second Edition*. (S. R. Meyers, Ed.) Chicago: American Dietetic Association.

Arnold, L. (2006). The ethics of donor human milk banking. *Breastfeeding Medicine , 1* (1), 3-13.

Arnold, L. (2008). U.S. health policy and access to banked donor human milk. *Breastfeeding Medicine, 3*(4), 221-229.

Baumslag, N. (1995). *Milk, money and madness: The culture and politics of breastfeeding*. Santa Barbara, CA: Praeger.

FDA. (2010). *FDA working group backgrounder on banked human milk*. Retrieved from: http://www.fda.gov/downloads/AdvisoryCommittees/CommitteesMeetingMaterials/PediatricAdvisoryCommittee/UCM235642.pdf

FDA Update: FDA program advisory committee discusses safety of human milk banks. (2011). *AAP News, 32*(2). Retrieved from: http://aapnews.aappublications.org/content/32/2/6.1.full.pdf+html

References

FDA. (n.d.). *Compliance program guidance manual: Inspection of human cells, tissues and cellular and tissue-based products.* 7341.002. unsigned and undated

FDA. (2010). *Use of donor human milk.* Retrieved from: http://www.fda.gov/scienceresearch/specialtopics/pediatrictherapeuticsresearch/ucm235203.htm

FDA. (2014, February 10). *Current good manufacturing practices, quality control procedures, quality factors, notification requirements, and records and reports, for infant formula.* Docket No. FDA-1995-N-0036 (formerly 95N-0309)] .

Geddes, D.H.P. (2013). Preterm birth: Strategies for established adequate milk production and successful lactation. *Seminars in Fetal and Neonatal Medicine, 18*(3), 155-159.

HMBANA. (1990). *HMBANA position paper on donor human milk banking.* Retrieved from: https://www.hmbana.org/downloads/position-paper-safety-ethical.pdf

HMBANA. (2014). *About us.* Retrieved from: http://www.hmbana.org/hmbana-about

Human Milk 4 Human Babies. (2014). *Informed milksharing network.* Retrieved from: http://hm4hb.net

Ip, S., Chung, M., Raman, G., Chew, P., Magula, N., DeVine, D., Trikalinos, T., & Lau, J. (2007). *Breastfeeding and maternal and infant health outcomes in developed countries.* Evidence Report/Technology Assessment Number 153. AHRQ Publication No. 07-E007.

Jones, F. (2003). History of north american donor milk banking: One hundred years of progress. *Journal of Human Lactation, 19*, 313-318.

Miracle, D.J., Szucs, K.A., Torke, A.M., & Helft, P.R. (2011). Contemporary ethical issues in human milk-banking in the United States. *Pediatrics, 128*, 1186-1189.

Montagne, P., Cuilliere, M.L., Mole, C., Bene, M.C., & Faure, G. (1999). Immunological and nutritional composition of human milk in relation to prematurity and mother's parity during the first 2 weeks of lactation. *Journal of Pediatric Gastroenterology and Nutrition, 29*, 75-80.

Prolacta Bioscience. (2014). *Prolact+ H 2 MF Human Milk Fortifier.* Retrieved from: http://www.prolacta.com/human-milk-fortifier

Swanson, K. (2011). Body banks: A history of milk banks, blood banks, and sperm banks in the United States. *Enterprise and Society, 12*(4), 749-760. doi: 10.1093/es-3khr038, 749-759.

References

Tully, MR. (2002). Recipient prioritization and use of human milk in the hospital setting. *Journal of Human Lactation, 18*(4), 393-396.

Underwood, M.A. (2013). Human milk for the premature infant. *Pediatric Clinics of North America , 60,* 189-207.

World Health Organization. (2008). *Childhood overweight and obesity.* Retrieved from: http://www.who.int/dietphysicalactivity/childhood/en/

Chapter 8

Expanding and Improving Media Support for Breastfeeding

Glanz, K., Rimer, B.K., & Viswanath, K. (2008). (Eds.). *Health behavior and health education: Theory, research and practice.* 4th Ed. San Francisco: Jossey-Bass.

Khoury, A.J., Moazzem, S.W., Jarjoura, C.M., Carothers, C., & Hinton A. (2005). Breast-feeding initiation in low-income women: Role of attitudes, support, and perceived control. *Women's Health Issues, 15*(2), 64-72. doi: 10.1016/j.whi.2004.09.003.

Kloeblen, A.S., Thompson, N.J., & Miner, K.R. (1999). Predicting breast-feeding intention among low-income pregnant women: A comparison of two theoretical models. *Health Education & Behavior, 26*(5), 675-688.

Kools, E.J., Thijs, C., & de Vries, H. (2005). The behavioral determinants of breast-feeding in the Netherlands: Predictors for the initiation of breast-feeding. *Health Education & Behavior, 32*(6), 809-824. doi: 10.1177/1090198105277327.

Manstead, A.S., Proffitt, C., & Smart, J.L. (1983). Predicting and understanding mothers' infant-feeding intentions and behavior: Testing the theory of reasoned action. *Journal of Personality & Social Psychology, 44*(4), 657-671.

Sittlington, J., Stewart-Knox, B., Wright, M., Bradbury, I., & Scott, J.A. (2007). Infant-feeding attitudes of expectant mothers in Northern Ireland. *Health Education Research, 22*(4), 561-570. doi: 10.1093/her/cyl113.

Vari, P., Camburn, J., & Henly, S. (2000). Professionally mediated peer support and early breastfeeding success. *Journal of Perinatal Education, 9*(1), 22-30.

Williams, P.L., Innis, S.M., Vogel, A.M., & Stephen, L.J. (1999). Factors influencing infant feeding practices of mothers in Vancouver. *Canadian Journal of Public Health, 90*(2), 114-119.

Mediating Mother Support: Social Networks, Online Discussion, and Breastfeeding Support

Barak, A., Boniel-Nissim, M., & Suler, J. (2008). Fostering empowerment in online support groups. *Computers in Human Behavior, 24*(5), 1867-1883. doi:10.1016/j.chb.2008.02.004

References

Plantin, L., & Daneback, K. (2009). Parenthood, information, and support on the Internet. A literature review of research on parents and professionals online. *BMC Family Practice, 10:34*, 101-112. doi:10.1186/1471-2296-10-34

U.S. Department of Health and Human Services. (2011). *The Surgeon General's Call to Action to Support Breastfeeding.* Washington D.C.: U.S. Department of Health and Human Services, Office of the Surgeon General.

Portrayals and Representations of Infant Feeding Practices in Primetime U.S. Television Media: A Discourse Analysis

Ayres, L., Kavanaugh, K., & Knafl, K.A. (2003). Within-case and across case approaches to qualitative data analysis. *Qualitative Health Research, 13*(6), 871-883.

Bandura, A. (2004). Social cognitive theory for personal and social change by enabling media. In A. Singhal and M.J. Cody (Eds.), *Entertainment-education and social change: History, research, and practice* (pp. 75-96). New York: Routledge.

Bartky, S.L. (1990). *Femininity and domination: Studies in the phenomenology of oppression.* New York: Routledge.

Bentley, M. E., Dee, D. L., & Jensen, J. L. (2003). Breastfeeding among low income, African American women: power, beliefs and decision making. *Journal of Nutrition, 133*(1), 305S-309S.

Brown, J.D., & Peuchaud, S.R. (2008). Media and breastfeeding: Friend or foe? *International Breastfeeding Journal, 3,* 15.

Centers for Disease Control and Prevention, CDC. (2010). *Breastfeeding report card—United States.* Retrieved from: http://www.cdc.gov/breastfeeding/data/reportcard/reportcard2010.htm.

Eidelman, A. I., Schanler, R. J., Johnston, M., Landers, S., Noble, L., Szucs, K., & Viehmann, L. (2012). Breastfeeding and the use of human milk. *Pediatrics, 129*(3), e827-e841.

Fairclough, N. (2000). Critical analysis of media discourse. In S. Thornham, C. Bassett, and P. Marris (Eds.), *Media studies: A reader* (pp. 308-325). New York: New York University Press.

Foss, K. A. (2012). "That's not a beer bong. It's a breast pump!" Representations of breastfeeding in prime-time fictional television. *Health Communication,* (ahead-of-print), 1-12.

Foss, K.E., & Southwell, B. (2006). Infant feeding and the media: The relationship between Parents' Magazine content and breastfeeding, 1972-2000. *International Breastfeeding Journal, 1,* 10.

References

Frederickson, B.L., & Roberts, T. (1997). Objectification theory: Toward understanding women's lived experiences and mental health risks. *Psychology of Women Quarterly, 21,* 173-206.

Frerichs, L., Andsager, J.L., Campo, S., Aquilino, M., & Dyer, C.S. (2006). Framing breastfeeding and formula-feeding messages in popular U.S. magazines. *Women and Health,* 44(1), 95-118.

Henderson, L., Kitzinger, J., & Green, J. (2000). Representing infant feeding: Content analysis of British media portrayals of bottle feeding and breast feeding. *British Medical Journal, 321,* 1196-1198.

Van Dijk, T. A. (1997). Discourse as interaction in society. In T. A. van Dijk (Ed.), *Discourse as social interaction* (pp. 1–37). London: Sage.

Media Reactions to Breastfeeding: Reactions to Recent Headlines

Hausman, B. L. (2012). Feminism and breastfeeding: Rhetoric, ideology, and the material realities of women's lives. In P.H. Smith, M. Labbok, and B. Hausman (Eds.), *Beyond health, beyond choice: Breastfeeding constraints and realities.* New Brunswick, NJ: Rutgers University Press.

Defeating the Formula Death Star, One Tweet at a Time: Using Social Media to Advocate for the WHO Code

Abrahams, S. W. (2012). Milk and social media: Online communities and the International Code of Marketing of Breast-milk Substitutes. *Journal of Human Lactation, 28*(3), 400-406. doi: 10.1177/0890334412447080.

Babendure, J. B. (2012). *If YOU don't advocate for mothers and babies, who will?* Retrieved from: http://lactationmatters.org/2012/11/08/if-you-dont-advocate-for-mothers-babies-who-will/

Bartholomew, M., Schoppe-Sullivan, S., Glassman, M., Kamp Dush, C., & Sullivan, J. (2012). New parents' Facebook use at the transition to parenthood. *Family Relations, 61*, 455-469.

Escobar, N.O. (2013). *The International Code: Is it still relevant in an information age?* Retrieved from: http://lactationmatters.org/2013/03/12/the-international-code-part-1/

Friends of the WHO Code. (n.d.) *Friends of the WHO Code Facebook page.* Retrieved from: https://www.facebook.com/groups/friendsofthewhocode/

Forbes, B. (2011). *What is the WHO-CODE?* Retrieved from: http://www.bestforbabes.org/what-is-the-who-code

References

Fox, S., & Jones, S. (2009). *The social life of health information: Americans' pursuit of health takes place within a widening network of both online and offline sources.* Washington, DC: Pew Internet and American Life Project. Retrieved from: http://www.pewinternet.org/~/media/Files/Reports/2009/PIP_Health_2009.pdf.

Gerber Corporation. (n.d.) *Gerber Facebook page.* Retrieved from: www.facebook.com/Gerber.

Howe, N., Strauss, W., & Matson, R. J. (2000). *Millennials rising: The next great generation.* New York: Vintage Books.

Kvedar, J. C., & Kibbe, D.C. (2009). Building a research agenda for participatory medicine. *Journal of Participatory Medicine, 1*(1), e16.

La Leche League International. (n.d.) *Annual Report: 2010-2011.* Retrieved from: http://www.llli.org/docs/00000000000000001AnnualReport/llli_ar2011_final.pdf

Lenhart, A., Purcell, K., Smith, A., & Zickuhr, K. (2010). *Social media and mobile internet use among teens and young adults.* Washington, DC: Pew Internet & American Life Project. Retrieved from: http://web.pewinternet.org/~/media/Files/Reports/2010/PIP_Social_Media_and_Young_Adults_Report_Final_with_toplines.pdf.

Mettera, P. (2013). *Nestlé: Corporate rap sheet.* Retrieved from: http://www.corp-research.org/nestle

McCann, A. (2012). *Worldwide impact in 10 minutes or less: Using social media for powerful change*. Retrieved from: http://lactationmatters.org/2012/11/14/world-wide-impact-in-10-minutes-or-less-using-social-media-for-powerful-change-2/

Nestlé Corporation. (n.d.). *History*. Retrieved from: http://www.nestle.com/AboutUs/History

NestleCorporate. (2012). *Digital acceleration team* [Video file]. Retrieved from: https://www.youtube.com/watch?v=ktsMa8hfgY0.

Smith, A. (2012). *17% of cell phone owners do most of their online browsing on their phone, rather than a computer or other device*. Washington DC: Pew Internet and American Life Project. Retrieved from http://www.pewinternet.org/~/media/Files/Reports/2012/PIP_Cell_Phone_Internet_Access.pdf.

Stevens, H. (2011). Social media giving birth to new generation of parents-to-be. *Chicago Tribune*. Retrieved from: http://connect.mayoclinic.org/news-articles/863-social-media-giving-birth-to-new-generation-of-parents-to-be/portal

Thomasson, E. (2012). *Insight–at Nestlé, interacting with the online enemy*. Retrieved from: http://uk.reuters.com/article/2012/10/26/uk-nestle-online-water-idUKBRE89P07Q20121026

References

Van Grove, J. (2010). *Nestle meets Greenpeace's demands following social media backlash.* Retrieved from: http://mashable.com/2010/05/17/nestle-social-media-fallout/

World Health Organization. (1981). *International Code of Marketing of Breast-milk Substitutes.* Geneva: World Health Organization. Retrieved from: http://whqlibdoc.who.int/publications/9241541601.pdf

Made in the USA
Charleston, SC
03 September 2015